CREATE POSITIVE TRANSFORMATION IN
YOUR WELL-BEING, BUSINESS, AND LIFE

THE POWER OF
ESSENTIAL OILS

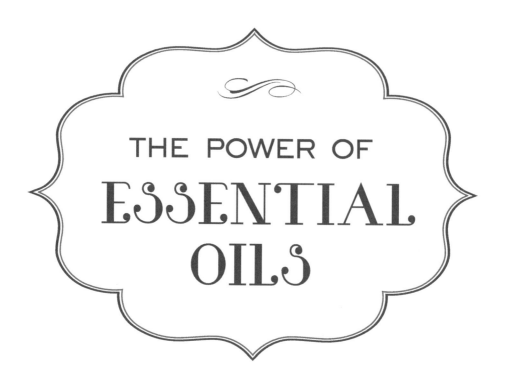

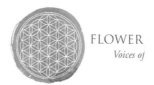

FLOWER
Voices of

D1445284

CONTENTS

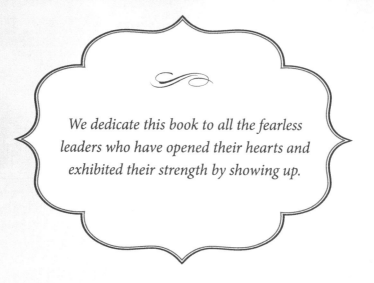

We dedicate this book to all the fearless leaders who have opened their hearts and exhibited their strength by showing up.

Proceeds from every Amazon sale are being donated to:

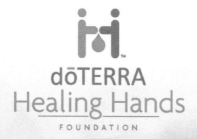

dōTERRA
Healing Hands
FOUNDATION

The dōTERRA˙ *Healing Hands Foundation* is dōTERRA International's registered 501(c)(3) non-profit organization committed to improving lives through partnering with organizations that offer hope to millions around the world. *Healing Hands* seeks to bring healing and hope to the world, for lives free of disease and poverty, and to ultimately empower impoverished communities with the tools needed to become self-reliant.

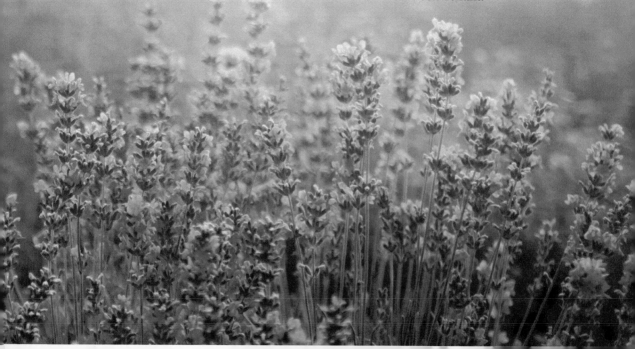

INTRODUCTION

by Jane Ashley, MA, CHHC

Publisher & dōTERRA Wellness Advocate

PASSION DRIVES US, FUELS OUR DREAMS, AND BRINGS POWER TO OUR **NOW!**

During my journey from girl to woman, the fire of passion has always been my guidepost—that feeling of excitement and power when something feels just right.

As my career unfolded and I learned more and more about natural solutions for health care, plants and their innate power became a bigger part of my life. When I put those first few drops of essential oil in the palms of my hands, I got that feeling, the *zing!* that says this stuff is special, and I want more.

As a book publisher, I look for ideas that will generate that passion in readers—as a mother and a coach, I know that essential oils bring more than just excitement and special scents. It's the miracle of how plants teach and serve us that really brings essential oils to a new level of passionate commitment for me. When I spoke with Hayley Hobson about the idea for this book you are holding in your hands, I knew in my heart that we could create something fantastic, a compendium of wisdom and insight that would make everyone proud.

What an inspiring process it has been to guide this book, an education for me—not just in the power of essential oils, but also in the magic of true leadership. The voices of the women in this book rise above the fray, telling stories and sharing truths, spreading the healing energy of positivity and purpose, while bringing the gifts of Mother Earth to as many people as possible. I am so very proud to bring this book to the world, and with the powerhouse women in this book standing with me, we will light that passionate flame for people everywhere.

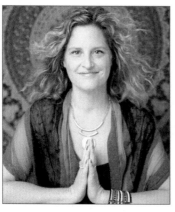

Jane Ashley, M.A., *wears many hats: wife and mom, artist and entrepreneur, transpersonal psychotherapist, dōTERRA wellness advocate, and health coach. Her passions come together when she is running her "other" company—as the Publisher of Flower of Life Press—where she produces brands and books that resonate with the Voices of Transformation, and supports her authors with holistic health resources. Jane knows the hurdles in launching a business, finding time for self-care, being with family and the importance of collaboration in this new economy. Her passion is to help women elevate their consciousness, lives, and businesses—by distilling their essence and creating a deep emotional connection through their message to a place they never dreamed possible, while breaking through perceived barriers to find joy and purpose in their lives. With the addition of two new imprints,* Ananda Art Books *and* Evolutionaries of Love, *Flower of Life Press now includes a home for artists and new paradigm leaders. Jane is a mom to five kids and lives with her family in Lyme, Connecticut.* **Learn more: www.FlowerofLifePress.com; Jane@FlowerofLifePress.com.**

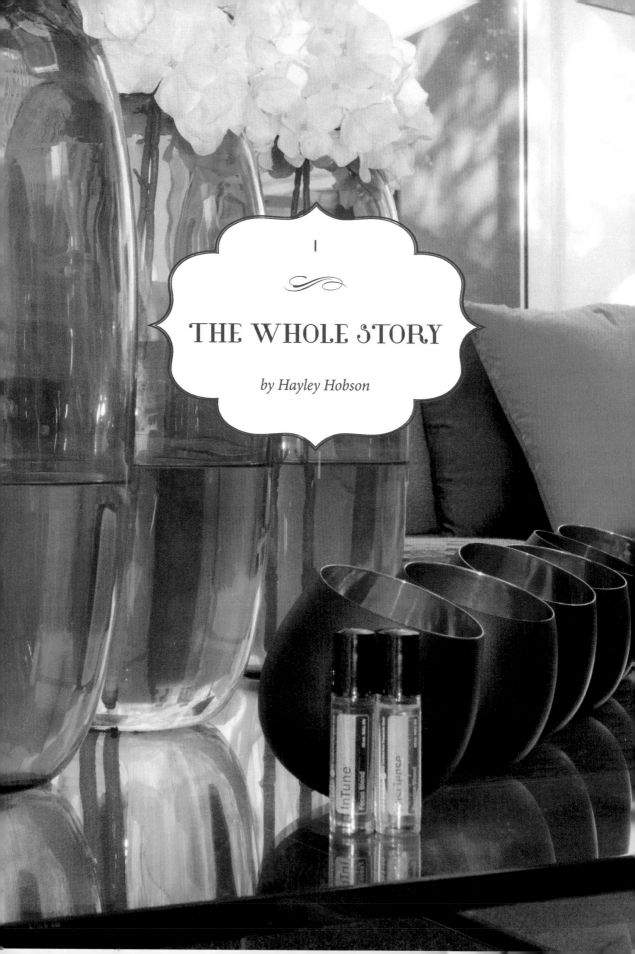

I

THE WHOLE STORY

by Hayley Hobson

I THOUGHT I HAD THE AMERICAN DREAM ALL FIGURED OUT. YOU GET A GOOD EDUCATION, SO YOU CAN GET A GOOD JOB, SO YOU CAN GET A GOOD PAYCHECK, AND THEN YOUR LIFE WILL JUST WORK.

So, I did that. And then five years into a very promising law career, I realized all I was doing was pushing paper from my desk to another lawyer's desk and back again. I thought as a lawyer I'd be helping people and be well compensated for it. And while I did make good money, most of it went to school loans, so I never really felt that I was getting anywhere financially. And I didn't seem to be making an impact.

I was always into health and fitness. Triathlon training was the thing that kept me sane through law school. And so, when I gave up law, I switched gears and went into health and fitness. Everyone, including my parents, thought I was crazy to give up the stable future they thought a law career would provide. But I knew law would never give me what I wanted. If I stayed in law, I'd burn out. I was *already* burnt out! I had been working 12-hour days and was left with nothing, not even a sense that I was doing good work. I quit and never looked back.

I built up my reputation as a yoga and Pilates instructor and found myself a few years later in Boulder, Colorado, with a full roster of private clients and managing a health club. There came a moment when I started to realize I was in the same situation as I was in the law firm. Yes, I was helping people transform their health and that felt good—really good. But I was still working 12-hour days. I still didn't feel like I was getting anywhere financially. I felt that my life was controlled by my clients. If I took a day off, I didn't make money. If someone canceled an appointment, I had to rebook them immediately or lose that money. While, on one level, I was satisfied, I was locked into this dollars-for-hours model that was no better than the weekly paycheck from the law firm.

Then I got sick.

Two years after the birth of my daughter, I was caught in this hamster wheel. Sure, I had my own business and set my own hours. But one last-minute cancellation could wreck my budget for the month. I was working harder and harder trying to divide my time between my family and my business. And my body just stopped working.

It was Christmas Day. On our eight-hour drive back to Boulder after visiting my in-laws, I threw up the whole way. My doctor put me on IV fluids, ran tests, and found nothing. In desperation, I went to see a natural doctor up in the Canyon. I'd heard a lot about him over the years and knew it was impossible to get an appointment. But I hadn't eaten anything in eight days, and he heard my desperation. He put me on his table, took my pulse, and said my body was in a state of total fight or flight and that all my organs were shutting down. I needed to change something about my life to save my life.

You would think that would be devastating news, but I burst into tears of relief. It was like I finally knew what was wrong, so now I could fix it. And what was wrong was my whole life.

This showed me that everything I knew about myself and what I wanted was wrong. Everything I knew about making money was wrong. And everything I knew about what "healthy" meant was wrong.

To live to see my daughter grow up, I had to find a way to be in control of my health, control of my time, and control of my money.

I started with my health. You would think as a yoga and Pilates instructor, I was pretty strong. And I was. But that didn't keep me from being sick. So I started taking precautionary measures, guarding myself from stress and inflammation by exercising daily but at more reasonable levels, getting quality sleep, and supporting my nutrition needs through a plant-based diet and juicing. I looked at toxins in my home and in the products I used and looked for natural solutions. In my mission to regain and protect my health, I used essential oils to support my immune system, to soothe sore muscles and joints, to encourage myself to relax, and to replace those chemical-laden products I had used—that nearly all of us used—in myriad ways, from skincare to cleaning products to artificial flavoring. I went from treating symptoms to supporting the various systems of my body—naturally.

The impact on my body was immediate and profound. But I also knew that if I didn't find a way to change my work, I'd find myself right back at the doctor's. Stress was rampant in my life, and stress is the number-one cause of disease. To eliminate some stress I took a leave of absence from work. I think it was the first time in my life that I was in 100 percent control of how I spent my time. I didn't have to show up on the clock to get paid, and I wasn't being held hostage to my clients' schedules. That break showed me that I had to find a way to make money completely on my terms.

I knew about the business-building opportunity with dōTERRA from the start. I had done some other Multi-Level Marketing (MLM) work in the past and had made a little bit of income with it. Network marketing seemed to me to be a lot of work for a little return. I didn't really understand the business model, and all my perceptions were off.

While I was on my leave of absence, I took a hard look at what I found most satisfying in the work I was doing. I stripped everything away and, at the core, I wanted to spend time helping other people. That was it. I was always at my best when I was helping people achieve their goals. If you were being successful as a direct result of working with me, that was when I was most fulfilled. That was the thing I could be passionate about and could put my energy into. I had to find a way to do that didn't have me putting in more time to make more money.

With that—helping people live better lives—as my foundation, I took a fresh look at dōTERRA. I knew the products helped me stay healthy. Every person who I gave oils to saw the benefits somewhere in their lives. What could this business opportunity look like if I focused solely on helping my team achieve their goals? When done right, that is what network marketing is about.

I started focusing on my team and what they needed to be successful. We talked about their goals, what's stopping them, what skills did they need to live the lives that they want. The more successful my team was, the more successful I would be.

As I started working with more and more people, I heard the same stories over and over.

People are stressed out, they're drowning in toxic chemicals, and the "healthcare" system tends to get involved when health breaks down. We're working harder than ever, and families are stretched thin with time and money. We're trained throughout our lives that the only way to make more money is to work more. Also, somewhere along the way we internalize that wanting to make more money is somehow bad or that we're not worthy of having more. This, your mindset around money, might be the thing that keeps you from having all of your financial needs taken care of. Time and again, when I talk to people about starting their own business and working with essential oils, I hear an undercurrent of "I don't deserve it." Or that making money is somehow bad. In the yoga community, it's almost shameful if you say you want to have a six-figure business. Sometimes I hear "It's too hard" and other similar excuses.

Do I work hard? Yes! But is the work hard? No. The biggest benefit in working with a network marketing company is that you have all the tools you need to be successful and community to help you do it. If you're not making the kind of income you want with your business—or even your 9-to-5 corporate job—your mindset needs a tune-up.

People ask me how I got successful. "Luck and hard work," I quip. But it was more than that. When I sat down and thought about what was underneath "luck and hard work," I saw there were five key things—things that anyone can replicate and use to produce results.

Five Factors for Success

1. I took control of my whole life, my health, my time, and my income.
2. I shifted my mindset about money and how to generate income.
3. I focused on my online presence and being known as a trusted expert.
4. I invested in the success of my team.
5. I got rid of all the excuses that had me settle for what was possible.

My success with my essential oil company is a direct result of the investment I have made with my team and myself and the work I've done around shifting my mindset with money. I get up every morning, and I push my excuses aside and focus on what is going to make our day, together as a team, successful. And I go to bed at night thankful that I have the ability to touch so many lives, thankful that I get to say how I live my whole life.

When I was introduced to essential oils, I was very excited about the power the products had to transform my health and wellbeing. I was less excited about the business opportunity because I knew I'd face an immediate challenge. Wes, my husband, summed it up pretty well when I told him that I was going to go all in with the business opportunity. "I don't know where you're going to sell it," he said. "Boulder is a really saturated market."

And he was right. Boulder, Colorado, is one of those strange places where you can't walk down the street without tripping over a wellness business. I was already running a thriving Pilates business here, and I knew introducing essential oils would do well. But competition would be fierce. To build the kind of business I wanted that could have a global impact, I knew from the very beginning, I would have to take my business online.

But here's the problem: I didn't want to be one of those people who was constantly spamming friends on Facebook with their "business opportunity" and products. I just didn't want to be that person who was always in your face trying to sell stuff. At the same time, I knew people were hungry for information about wellness. When I started creating my online presence, I focused mainly on branding and telling a good story.

Branding is creating a total picture of who you are and what you do as a business. It's not just a fancy logo or website design. I've nicknamed my brand the "Whole You." My brand looks at being holistically healthy in all areas of your life and, of course, essential oils are a vehicle that helps get you there. By focusing on the Whole You concept, I can talk about exercise, diet, and other aspects of health and how they are supported by essential oils. But I can also talk about career and money, as you can't be holistically healthy if you are in a job you hate forty hours a week or more.

Good branding takes the pressure off selling product. It's just part of the story and a natural conclusion to the conversation. Good branding seeks to solve a problem, not just sell a product. And you need good branding if you're going to operate online. Let's face it, you can only say "Buy my stuff" so many times before people stop listening to you.

If you want to create a brand around your business, look at these three things:

- What is your why? Why are you in business? Why are you passionate about these products?
- What problems does your audience face? How do you solve those problems?
- What's the emotional experience that you want your audience to have?

Almost everything I create online comes back to these three points. I share why I'm passionate about detoxing my home and my life. I blog about issues my audience deals with. And I am always seeking to do that in a fun and entertaining way.

Let's face it—many people do what you do. Thousands upon thousands of people work in your network marketing business. I don't like to use the word compete, but you are competing in a crowded market for attention from an audience. Why I don't like to use the word compete is that if you have a strong brand, there is no competition—you are the right solution for your target audience.

When you unlock your mindset around money and embrace branding, you can have amazing success with essential oils and network marketing.

When I look at what I created this past year, the thing I'm most proud about is that I created a seven-figure business. And there are six people on my team all set to hit the six-figure milestone in the coming year.

I cannot wait for the day when I can say, "I helped someone make a million dollars." Wow, I almost want to cry thinking about that!

This book is a tribute to women I have known over the past few years with dōTERRA. I truly believe that the single reason I have been successful in this business is because I have invested in the success of others. Success breeds success. Sharing these powerful stories is not a pat on the back for us. Consider this a tool for you to see what's possible for you.

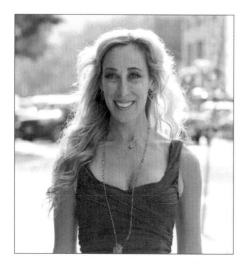

Hayley Hobson is an author, speaker, mentor, business coach, mom, and entrepreneur. She began her career as a bankruptcy attorney and quickly moved into entertainment law. After several years in law, she made the bold move to pursue her passion: health and wellness. Hayley knew she could have a bigger impact on people's lives as a health coach than she ever could as a lawyer. She relocated to Boulder, Colorado, and managed several fitness studios and built a thriving Pilates and yoga business with a full client roster. Three years ago, Hayley added essential oils to her business and broke company records by achieving Double Blue Diamond status in under 26 months and then Presidential Diamond in 3 years. She now holds the rank of Double Presidential Diamond. She travels extensively, educating people on how to improve their health and wellness by detoxing and creating holistic health in all areas of their lives by including essential oils. She is also the creator of "The Social Downline," a program teaching other network marketers how to build their business online, Your "Whole Biz," a business education course for network marketers, and "Six-Figure Moms," a community to support women in creating financial freedom. Learn more: www.HayleyHobson.com.

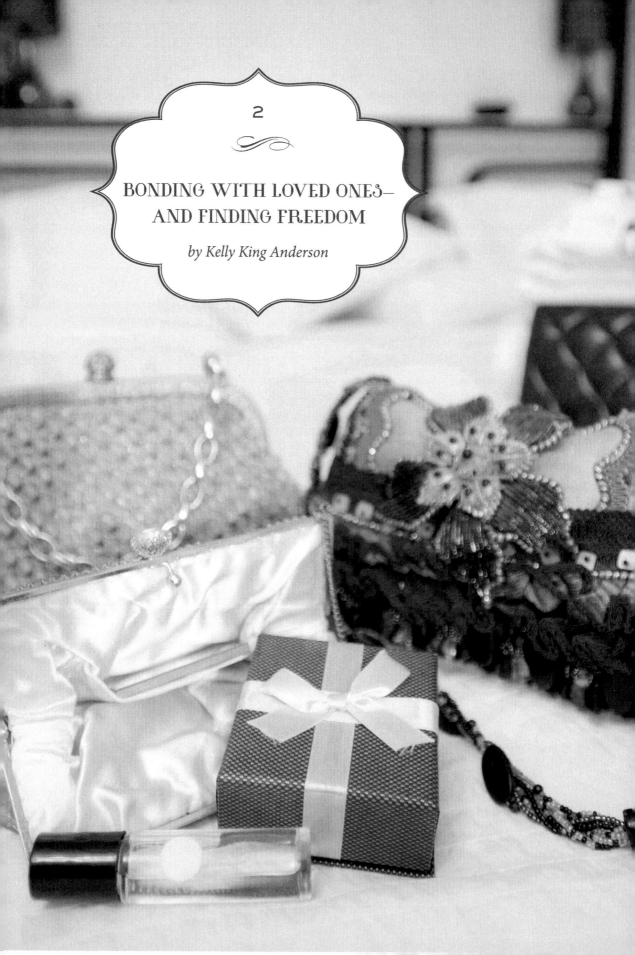

2

BONDING WITH LOVED ONES— AND FINDING FREEDOM

by Kelly King Anderson

OVER THE YEARS, ESSENTIAL OILS HAVE BECOME A LOVE LANGUAGE FOR OUR FAMILY. WHEN MY DAUGHTER WAS A BABY WE STARTED TO USE A DIFFUSER WITH CITRUS OILS TO CALM HER AND IT BECAME A CHERISHED ROUTINE FOR OUR FAMILY.

If my daughter would start to cry her brother, aged four at the time, would say, "Mommy! She needs her oils!" Then we would get out the oils and she would be smiling once again.

We noticed a remarkable difference with the mood in our home as we used the oils topically as well. We all like to have little massages with oils regularly, and it has now become one of the most precious moments of our day. As my husband and I take the time to connect with our children by applying oils on them it gives us a chance to talk and help them to relax before bedtime. For a while, our teenage son resisted using oils because he didn't like how some of them smelled. But he recently gave me a card for Christmas that gave me "permission to use the oils on him whenever I wanted" because he has seen their effectiveness. He now joins his sisters in our nightly oil routine. It is so wonderful to see those who resist open up to the possibilities of wellness and see their benefits.

I am so grateful for our treasure box of oils that has increased family bonding not only for us but for millions around the world. Whenever I hear of a mother who enjoys massaging her child with oils I feel an immediate bond with her because we share something in common, a way of communicating love and nurturing that was not previously available to us as children, as if we've unlocked a secret of the universe.

Another secret of the universe that was unlocked to me was the oil business opportunity. Actually, it took a lot of patience from my friend Natalie to help me to be open to the idea. It was clear that dōTERRA offered a tremendous difference in quality compared to other brands. But I never considered it was part of my life purpose to sell them. In fact, I did not open a Wellness Advocate account, as I didn't want to be a part of one of "those" types of multi-level marketing companies. I just bought what I needed from my friend, and was content with that. I had such a negative attitude regarding network marketing that several times I passed up her offer to participate, nearly missing the gift that eventually changed our lives. Ironically, at the time I was a business coach actively looking for financial opportunities so we could realize our dreams of traveling worldwide as a family, serving a mission for our church, and being financially free. Yet I resisted the idea that the resources might show up in the form of an oil bottle! I was so afraid to be known as a "network marketer."

Then eighteen months later I had a massive mental shift when I was driving down the street admiring a gorgeous home for sale that I knew we could not afford. I realized in that moment that I was limiting our bank account because of my resistance to receiving abundance. At the time I held a core belief that money could flow only through a traditional exchanging hours-for-dollars business model. I started to pray about how abundance could be possible for our family, not because I wanted a gorgeous house but because I wanted more choices. I felt that there was more waiting for us to experience, particularly with volunteer service. I chose to take proactive steps to change our financial situation and sought advice from others who were generating multiple streams of income. Eventually I was ready and open to say yes to the oils business largely because I trusted that if it could work for my friend Natalie, I hoped it could work for me, too. For a while I was still hesitant to tell people I had joined a network marketing company. But as I saw that people loved using our product and that getting it for wholesale was the best deal for them, I started to gain more confidence in the business opportunity and I realized what I had been missing out on.

With the help of our inspiring friends and mentors Natalie and Andy Goddard and our wonderful, passionate team who is so committed and driven to share, we have been fortunate to create a strong thriving business that has since released us from financial concerns. We can work with whomever we want, when, how, and where we want, and no one limits what we can create. I now think network marketing is the best business plan in the world! Plus, there is so much gratitude considering we are helping families connect in meaningful ways as they care for one another.

Within two years of starting to build our business, my husband was able to retire, and, almost immediately, we were invited by our church to serve a volunteer mission as Entrepreneurs in Residence at Brigham Young University–Hawaii. We wouldn't have been able to accept this wonderful opportunity without our residual income. We have also realized our dream to travel extensively with our children all over Europe, Australia, New Zealand, and Asia, including a year abroad in Bali, Indonesia and six months in the charming beach town of Sayulita, Mexico, where we helped our team to expand to a new market.

I'm patient when the people I share oils with express concerns about network marketing, because that is how I felt before I knew what an empowering, liberating business opportunity had been presented to me. I tell them they are welcome to buy the oils at retail just I like I did initially or they can get a membership account right away and save a significant amount of money. I also let them know that by consistently sharing the oils that have blessed their lives with others, they too can begin to make their greatest dreams a reality. It is such a win to help families to draw closer and be financially rewarded, a joy that doesn't even feel like work! With faith, focused effort, passion, and belief in the process, anything is possible. I am so happy and grateful to be a part of this special opportunity and share it with others looking to create a meaningful change in their lives.

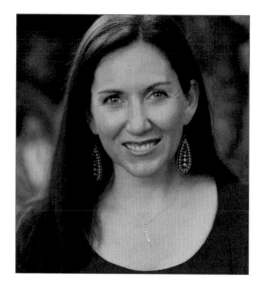

Kelly King Anderson loves to inspire others to create their dreams by faith, hard work, and solid mentoring. In addition to her team mentoring, Kelly coached for several years with her award-winning organization for women, Startup Princess, as an Entrepreneur in Residence at BYU Hawaii, and with her Creating with God Project. Kelly, her husband Matthew, and three children enjoy the flexible lifestyle of residual income and the blessed opportunity of working and serving wherever they choose. Recently they spent a year in Bali, Indonesia and then at the beach for six months in Sayulita, Mexico, where they were supporting new dōTERRA leaders. They now live in the beautiful mountains of Heber, Utah. Kelly and Matthew are Presidential Diamonds. Learn more: www.6weekstosilver.com.

THOUGHTS ON
LEADERSHIP

by Kelly King Anderson

Are you constantly trying to squeeze in time to work whenever possible—lunch breaks, nap times, or whenever the house is quiet? I get it! When I started, I had little kids and another business to run so I declared that I would build by faith, quickly and easily. No one wants to grow the long and slow way! I'm happy to share my best tips that have made all the difference for moving at a steady, smooth pace and staying on target for each of my ranks.

My first recommendation is to get into your heart each day before you begin and ponder how your time can best be spent. Ask who is ready and open to share the oils, that you might be led to them first. I would rather our conversations be with people who are ready to share our products and opportunity than connecting with people who will only keep it to themselves. When we get to those who will open their mouths our time and energy is maximized. Try this mantra as part of your daily personal development affirmations, "A key to my success is enrolling leaders who enroll leaders."

Your leaders need to be discovered and served; they are waiting for you! How do you find leaders who enroll? They are the influencers in your community on or offline. They are often already a business owner or actively supporting causes as a volunteer. These are people you might even be nervous to talk to, because you admire them so much! If this is the case, please talk to your mentor and create a plan on how to best approach them and invite them to experience the oils.

Don't be surprised if this sort of leader needs time to enroll; they are worth the effort and they likely will not sign up during the first conversation or even second. Can you share your diffuser with them for a week? Give them an intro kit as a thank you gift? They will do their research on you, the company, and the product—and you want them to! When they do, they will find that it all checks out because of the integrity and quality we offer, and you will have your next leader who enrolls leaders! As we all know, this sort of leader becomes a Diamond.

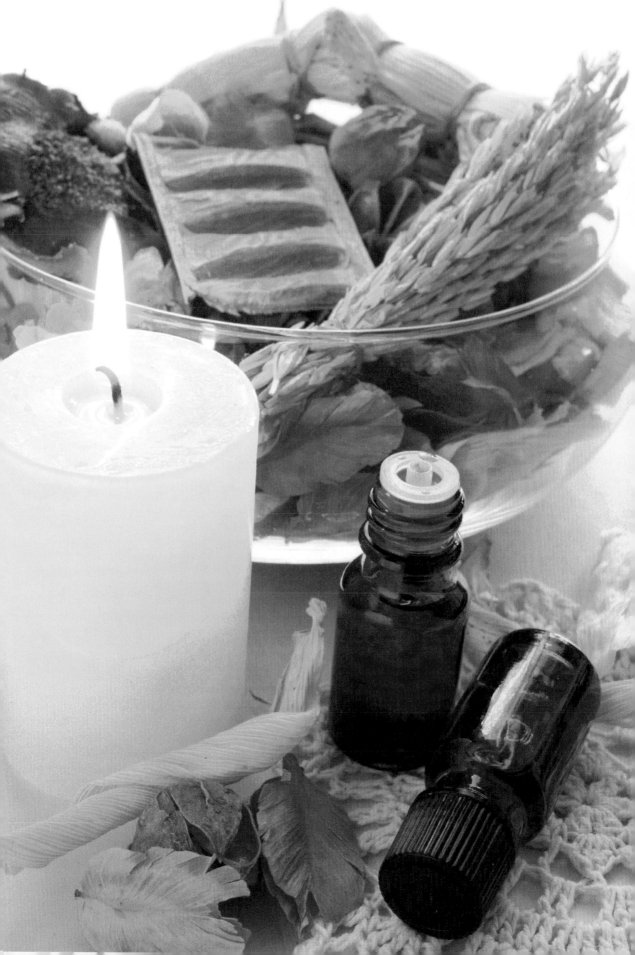

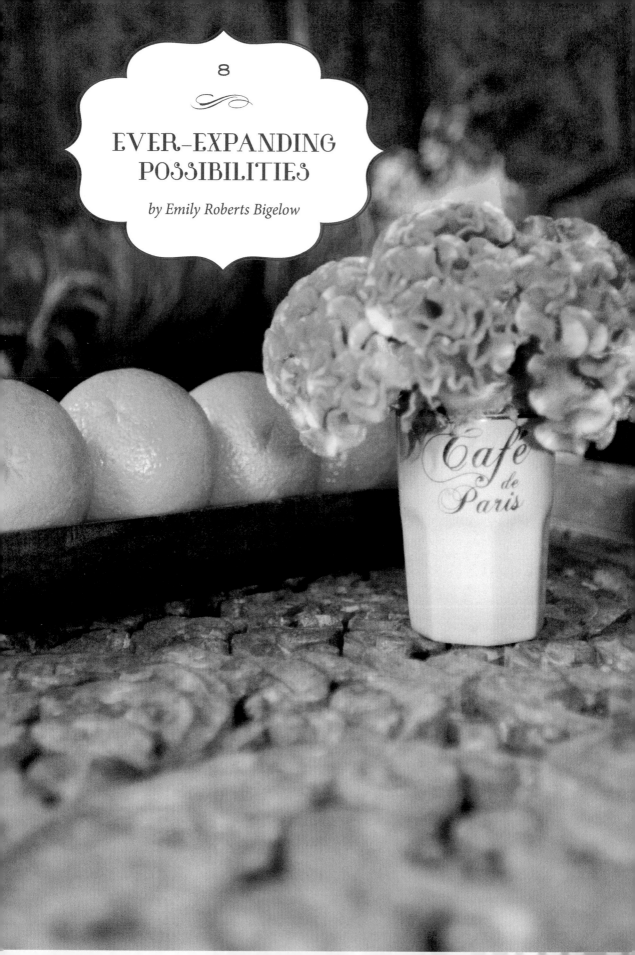

8

EVER–EXPANDING POSSIBILITIES

by Emily Roberts Bigelow

I STARTED MY ADULT LIFE ENTIRELY TOO EARLY. I WAS A BABY WHO HAD A
BABY. I BUCKLED DOWN, FINISHED HIGH SCHOOL A YEAR BEFORE MY CLASS,
AND OFF TO FULL TIME WORK I WENT AS A SINGLE MOTHER.

Long sporadic work hours spent in management at a large retail chain meant the same long sporadic hours for daycare at less than desirable "open early and late" facilities, the effects of which reached far into the depths of our lives. I firmly believe: Everything affects everything.

Twelve years later, the blending of two families eventually allowed me to create a "stay"-at-home momma lifestyle that was really a "work"-at-home lifestyle. I threw myself into caring for the children and responding to their every need. Seven years flew by, and the children were developing lives of their own. I began to feel the left-behind fragments of who I was and started to piece together what I wanted, who I was, and how I wanted to direct my future from here. Sure, I had done and accomplished "things" all those years, but I realized I had lost or given up quite a bit of me in the process. I wasn't sure who I was or what I wanted, and I didn't even know what I liked to do. Really, if I was given a week care-free, what would I want to do with my all time?

When my grandmother passed away, I read in her journal that she regretted not keeping in better contact with her friends. I realized I had been so busy tending to mom tasks that I hadn't really been a friend. A considered the adage: "To have a friend, be a friend." Not only did I not know who I was or what I liked, but I hadn't been a good friend, and didn't have many great friends. To top that off, I had been out of the "workforce" for seven years and was left wondering where I could or would want to jump back in if I had the opportunity. We really do weigh heavily our contribution to society. Ouch, salt on a wound.

I didn't set out to be a leader. I was invited to a class, and because there wasn't much else to do on that dark Alaskan evening, I attended. I hadn't a clue really what "essential oils" were. But I went, I listened, and I smelled. I didn't buy. I didn't know where to begin with those "things."

But my curiosity was sparked, and so I did some more research and placed an order. I kept my oils handy and put them to work. I tried them on every chance I had. Time and again the oils were helpful. I shared with a friend and what do you think happened? She wanted some. I didn't know how exactly, but we figured out how to get her an account, too. A week or so went by and I got a check in the mail. Wow, cool. Wait, Wow, cool! I share with a friend, and I get a check. Really?

By then, the oils were becoming my norm. I decided to bring the oils to my mom to share them with her. I left her with a Family Physician's Kit™ with a little info so she would know how to use what. A couple days later she called me, and with an inflection in her voice like a high school girl calling her bestie after a hot date, she said, "Emily! You have to tell people about those oils! That Deep Blue® is amazing and if you knew what I know, if you've seen what I've seen, YOU HAVE TO TELL PEOPLE ABOUT THOSE OILS."

That was one of the many miracle seeds planted along my path as I walked further and further on my journey. The time was right, and the conditions were right. I was ready to contribute, to help others, to get out socially, and to earn my own income again.

In my experience, if given the choice, most people would rather take the healthier, more natural route. They just don't know with what or how to do that. I decided I would open my mouth and just share. So I did, and I quickly found myself in constant conversations; whether they were ready or not, I would tell them. And tell them I did. Again and again and again.

I watched webinars, read books, and listened to podcasts and audio CDs about network marketing, health, and wellness as a whole. Then I put the information I learned to practice. I kept sharing, kept enrolling, kept having meetings, and kept getting people together. Over and over and over. It grew. *I* grew. I was a sponge learning as much as I could about sales, communication, leadership, the mind, goal setting, oils—everything I could get my hands on.

What did that do? It has, over the last few years, put me on the path with some incredible people. I can't imagine I would have ever met them were it not for my company, and I can't imagine my life without them. They richly bless my life just by knowing them and their stories! This adds fuel to my fire, reminds me of my purpose to contribute, to help, to make a difference, to share with those who just don't know yet that there is a healthier, more natural way.

This journey has driven me to personally know more and do better, mentally and physically. I am not the same woman who started this journey. Now, I think before I speak, and I listen intently. I try to understand that everyone is fighting a battle we know nothing of, but if you will make time to listen, they will share with you. There are ways we can help each other. That is what we were sent here to do.

I have learned, sacrificed, and shared relentlessly at times. The oils are what I do; they are in everything I do. And what have the oils done for me? I now know who I am, what I like, what drives me, and what I can contribute. Because of the oils, I have created a richly abundant life full of love, caring, knowledge, and wealth. They have inspired me and others to dream bigger and clearer—to open up to new, ever-expanding possibilities.

Everything affects everything. Years ago I might not have known what I would have done with a week. Now, the possibilities are endless!

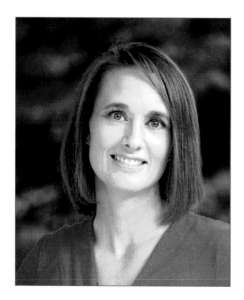

Emily Roberts Bigelow joined in 2010 and was one of the first 100 Wellness Advocates to achieve Diamond. Not starting dōTERRA as a business changed as she realized she needed to share this message of hope, health, and healing. Emily's passion for natural wellness fuels her lifestyle of nutrition and fitness. She is currently studying at the Institute of Integrative Nutrition. Her personal mission is to "To serve, inspire, and to teach, thereby changing one life at a time, physically, emotionally, and financially leaving the world a better place." **Learn more: www. bethebig.com; beyourtribe@gmail.com.**

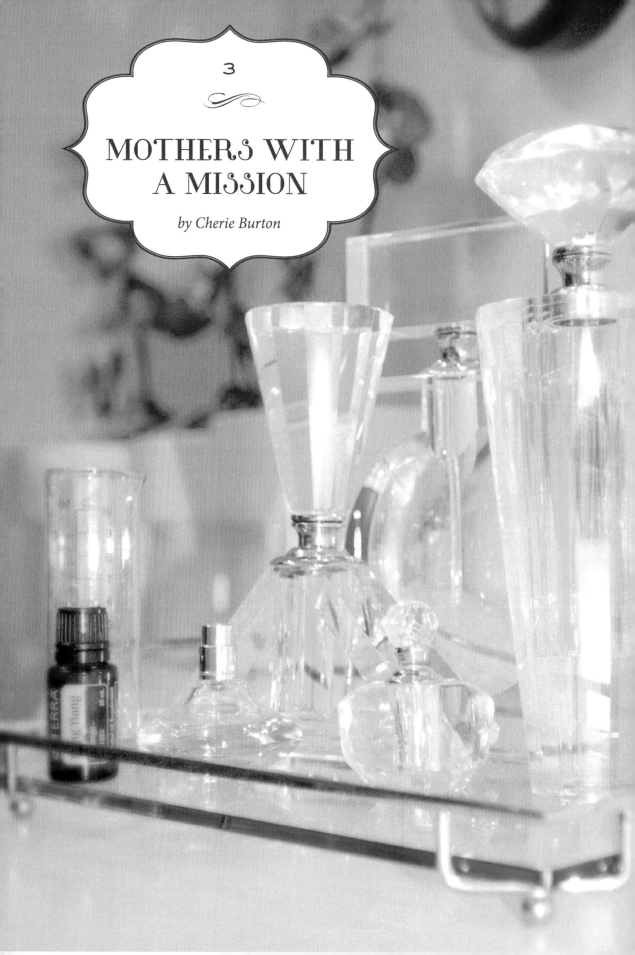

3

MOTHERS WITH A MISSION

by Cherie Burton

At one point in my upbringing, my family lived in a single-wide trailer with five children. My dad was a policeman and worked hard to provide. Mom used her skills in resourceful ways to add to the family income. She was entrepreneurial, but back then, the word hardly existed in the marketplace, much less for a stay-at-home mother. She delivered newspapers, sewed wedding dresses, baked homemade bread and sold it, and even took my sisters and I with her to clean bathrooms at the local high school when I was ten. At that young age, I remember thinking, "My mama wasn't born to clean other people's toilets, and *neither am I!*" And that trailer we were living in? Not our destiny, not what we were born for.

Despite our impoverished circumstances, my parents instilled within me a work ethic and mindset that refused to think prosperity was reserved for "other people." My mother would always remind me that my birthright was tied into this fancy word "abundance" and that I had a mission on this earth to fulfill. Over the years, I've learned abundance has little to do with materialism. Rather, it is a "*there is enough*" and an "*I am enough*" mentality. A person may be abundant *spiritually* but "lack" *physically*—riddled with health or body-image issues. Someone might have *financial wealth* but be lacking in the "others" department, struggling with loneliness or with maintaining intimacy in relationships. You can have someone who has very full, abundant relationships but they're lacking in *resources*—they're poor; they're in debt or can't cover living expenses. Why have wealth without health or without having strong relationships to enjoy your bounties with? Quoting a biblical reference: "What does it profit a man if he gains the whole world and loses his own *soul?*" Why have wealth if you lose your core identity and purpose?

From the time I was a young girl, I dreamed of having many children, in a big, beautiful home with a loving husband, helping people by being a teacher and writing books. That is what I *knew* I wanted—at the soul level—what I dreamed of and pined for, well into adulthood. As I matured, I had groups and causes I wanted to share my future abundance with. I wanted to have more so I could give more, sharing not only wealth but *knowledge*.

And then I became a mother.

I remember being eight months pregnant with our first baby, waddling around the halls of the psychiatric hospital where I worked, kind of avoiding processing the massive life shift about to hit me. Some patients would ask, "So, what are you going to do after the baby is born?" This was an internal conflict, trying to figure out how I was going to do motherhood alongside a life mission that had been calling to me for as long as I could remember. I wondered, *Can't I do what I love and still be an exceptional mom?* Many mothers are purpose-driven and wish to have an impact by doing something they're passionate about, something that inspires or—heaven forbid—creates *income*. I struggled with my heart's desire to have influence beyond my roles at home. I felt like I might be selling out on my kids, somehow jilting them by building a business or pursuing a passion. It took a shake-up in the dynamics of the family for me to come to terms with the lies that Mother Guilt perpetuates with ambitious women.

My husband, Jeff, became very successful with land development and real estate during the home building boom. But when the real estate market crashed, we lost everything, almost overnight. I was introduced to essential oils around this time and began casually sharing the oils with friends and clients, not in an effort to create income but because I was so fascinated by the oils. I began heavily researching the science behind these complex chemical compounds: how they work on the cellular level, the calming and relaxing effect they can have, and their unique ability to impact body chemistry.

A year after our financial crisis, my mom and sisters and I attended a dōTERRA convention. We came with the intent to learn more about the oils we'd grown to love but left with something we hadn't expected. At precisely the same moment, my sister Robin and I looked at each other across the table and said, "We need to start teaching other mothers about this." A sister pact was made between us that we would align with this special education-based wellness company and grow an organization focused on abundance on *all* levels. We have never looked back! With dedication and hard work, our outreach efforts have grown to a worldwide organization of many thousands strong, providing the opportunity to educate audiences throughout Australia, Asia, and North America.

Jeff left a job—one he was going through the motions with to provide for the family after the real estate crash—and joined me at home full-time in 2011 in our thriving business as new dōTERRA Diamonds. We've added two children to the three we had at that time and are now the rank of Blue Diamond. Honestly, we wouldn't even have these last two children without our miraculous journey in dōTERRA—the lessons learned, people met, health sustained, and finances healed.

If we listen closely to our children, we will discover that they are the ones who actually hold the deeper answers for our paths in life. In one breath our children are crying, "Mom, don't leave me" and in the next, "Show me how to live." *Show me how to lead, Mom. Give me permission to play full out in my life.* My kids know I *have* to do this; I simply *have* to teach. But they also know that in my heart, they are first— no question. It was my oldest child Noah, not my sister Robin, who was actually the first to say back in 2010, "Mom, you should share this with other moms." His simple statement sent shivers up my spine and gave me a special kind of permission. He is the one I was waddling around carrying as I worked in the psych hospital and faced my first existential crisis as a woman of purpose. And he is the one who now, as an eighteen-year-old high school grad, ventures out to fulfill his *own*. This son beams to everyone he knows that his parents are leaders of a global business that helps a lot of people. This son sits up with me late at night and talks to me about love and life and leadership. We both marvel at the miracles and adventures we've been part of and the beautiful and broken people who have come in and out of our doors.

In the big picture, it seems counterproductive and inconsequential to hold some Mother Guilt paradigm that I have somehow harmed him and the other kids by my zeal for connecting, sharing, and teaching.

Back when I was pursuing my psych degree, I thought about becoming a family therapist on a schedule that could somehow complement motherhood. What I'm doing now as a leader in dōTERRA, I believe, is farther reaching, more financially rewarding, and much more fulfilling. Because of the residual income business model, I have time to do the things that mean most to me: nurture my family, teach, and write: *exactly* what I wanted as a young girl. I see my business as sort of a personal ministry. My family, my church and community work, my friends, and my dōTERRA business are one big service mission to me. Their boundaries enmesh. This helps me to see things not from lack but from abundance: that I'm not taking away from one area to nurture another. I'm not taking away from my family to run a business. I'm not taking away from my business to run my family. I'm not taking away from my church responsibilities to run my home or my business. They are all one, and they are all *me*.

I love Marianne Williamson's quote: "Purity of heart is the greatest engine of wealth creation." As we shift our thinking to believing that we are *enough*—filling our minds and hearts with information that supports the belief that there is enough for *everyone*—our vision as leaders expands, and we help others step into their soul's true purpose. Jeff and I are on target to hit the rank of Presidential Diamond in dōTERRA soon. This rank is special to us not just because of the monetary compensation but because we have been able to help a number of very special people claim freedom. This company offers myself and other mothers a platform to not only build a business without unnecessarily sacrificing that sacred time with our families but to break generational patterns and build authentic confidence as leaders through genuine service.

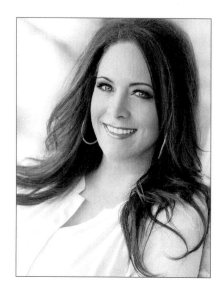

Cherie Burton is a mother of five who is passionately driven to help others find wholeness. She holds degrees in psychology and sociology and was a group therapist at various psychiatric facilities and an addiction recovery center. Cherie was Mrs. Utah 2004 and finds joy as an image, business, and life coach for women. She and her husband, Jeff, are Blue Diamonds in dōTERRA and travel the globe sharing natural solutions for families. Her upcoming book on emotional wellness is the culminating work of more than twenty years of extensive research and in-the-trenches outreach. Wellness, Beauty, Wholeness is the signature theme of her business. **Learn more: www.CherieBurton.com.**

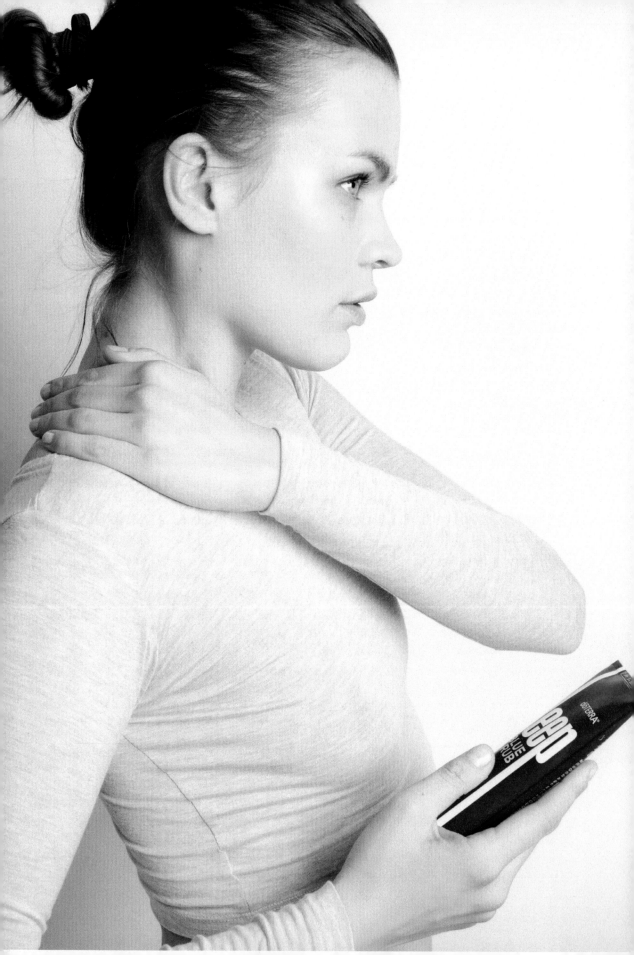

THOUGHTS ON
LEADERSHIP

by Cherie Burton

I think we unnecessarily complicate business because we try too hard to do what doesn't come naturally to us. I have learned to focus mostly on doing what I shine at: teaching and inspiring. The rest, I delegate to my husband, my team leaders, and my support staff. I can typically find someone who absolutely loves doing what I don't want to do and they are a thousand times better at it. A powerful value exchange happens when you meet others in the middle like that, and growth happens more authentically.

Certainty is what people crave when it comes to their health and prosperity. If you can stand in front of a group and proclaim, "I know I have solutions for you," they will be drawn to learn from you, be part of your movement.

Consistency is everything. If I have an idea, I owe it to myself to see it through. I am consistent and I feel like people can count on that consistency to support them, whether it is health or business needs.

Honest communication is crucial in business partnerships. I know if someone is serious about creation and has a business focus if they stay with me, energetically. As they disengage from regular rapport, I know they've disengaged from not only their business but also from their core desires and dreams. My role is to hold form for what they told me they wanted and to keep it honest and real.

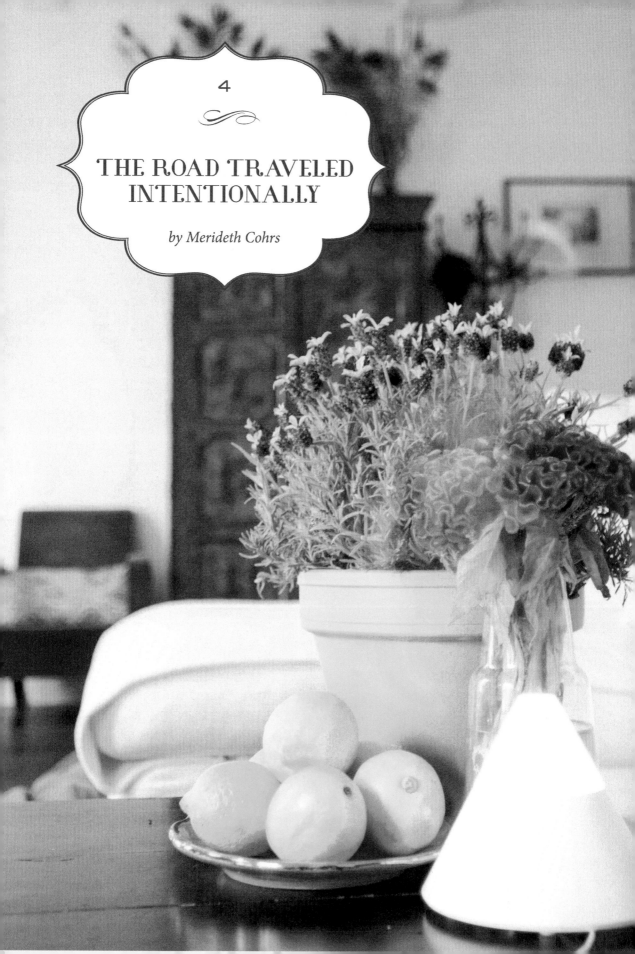

4

THE ROAD TRAVELED INTENTIONALLY

by Merideth Cohrs

"Two roads diverged in a wood, and I—
I took the one less traveled by,
And that has made all the difference."

—Robert Frost

<small>AS A YOUNG WOMAN, I LOVED ROBERT FROST'S POEM "THE ROAD NOT TRAVELED." I HAD A DEEP DESIRE TO CHOOSE THE ROAD THAT "MADE ALL THE DIFFERENCE" AND AT DIFFERENT TIMES IN MY LIFE THAT HAS MEANT DIFFERENT THINGS.</small>

My decision to pursue an appointment at the United States Naval Academy at the age of seventeen was the first decision of my life with the significance implied by Frost's poem. Confident, inspired, and fearless, I submitted my application to this prestigious institution and scoffed at the notion of building a back-up plan with a different school. I knew what I wanted and was going to do whatever it took to achieve my dream—a plan B would only be a distraction. Because of that single decision, I experienced the unique challenges of life as a Midshipman, traveled the world, served my country in a time of war, thrived in near-constant leadership challenges, and matured very quickly. I took great pride in my accomplishments and imagined they were a measure of my inherent ability to live life on my terms.

I married the love of my life at twenty-five, left the Navy at twenty-eight, and followed many of my peers into the corporate ranks with a respected federal government management consultancy firm. I achieved a six-figure salary, lived in a five-bedroom house, and had a "perfect" marriage. The birth of my son in 2009 and my smooth transition into the corporate world cemented my belief that I was living the American dream and that I was on the right path. I truly thought I had discovered the perfect formula for success. As a Naval Officer, I had learned to be a leader and a decision-maker unafraid to take action. As a consultant, I leveraged those skills as a polished expert. As a wife and mother, I made the right food, had the right house, and believed I was capable of "helping" the people around me be "perfect" as well. Despite how my life appeared, on the inside, I was intensely unhappy. The pressures of maintaining rigid control over my environment wore heavily on me and, ever so slowly, I felt the wheels begin to come off.

For me, change often happens at the speed of pain. The pain eventually became great enough to motivate massive action, and I came through the tumultuousness of that time changed for the better. I realized that the dreams, tenets, and ideals of my youth were simply not possible in a life where success was measured by standards that were not my own. I was walking down a path that someone else had carved. It was not easy and it was not mine.

While I could love and appreciate my wonderful and amazing family, being a wife and mother no longer singularly defined me. I needed to provide income to pay the bills, but I no longer had to do so in a manner that was dictated solely by others' expectations of what I "supposed" to do. I needed to do something that was authentic and reflected who I was. Merideth, the woman, began to emerge and I began to forge a new path. I decided it was time to start a business—a dream that had been tucked away inside me for quite some time.

With no experience to speak of, I pursued the path of entrepreneurship and learned to craft artisan truffles and confections. Within two years I was, by all accounts, a very successful business owner. My business, MC2 Confections, was profitable and I was a recognized leader and creative innovator throughout the region where I lived. But this success came with a heavy toll. Work was constant—nights, weekends, and every holiday were simply more hours to fill—with the result that I frequently missed key family moments. My son's first three years, my mother-in-law's struggle with cancer and her passing, and the simple celebration and enjoyment of life were lost to me. Looking back on this time, my heart breaks for the choices I made that prioritized my business over my family. It amazes me that my family didn't implode from the pressures and expectations.

Once again, my desire to change was proportional to the level of pain I experienced. But it was not the pain of missed family moments that ultimately pushed me over the edge—it was physical pain. Two years into my life as a business owner, I was exhausted and sick. I was ill, like clockwork, every two months. I ran my body hot, and the only time I let it come down was when I was "forced" down. I looked healthy on the outside, but I was running on fumes and very unhealthy on the inside. I began to develop severe pain and inflammation in my fingers and joints, and as it advanced, there came a time when I literally could not hold a pen to write a grocery list without intense difficulty. With a diagnosis of a chronic, progressive disease, I finally took notice of what I had been doing to my body.

I was once again provided with an opportunity to see that my current path was not going to result in the life I wanted. I was no longer willing to work seventy hours a week and accept that I had to sacrifice my body, mind, and spirit to achieve my goals. I was no longer willing to tell my son that I couldn't play with him because, "Mommy has to work." I was no longer willing to be roommates with my husband because I was too exhausted and stressed out for intimacy.

In my pursuit of happiness—true happiness—I began to look for a different way of taking care of my body, a different way of doing business, and a different way of being. This required a lot of change including some massive development of my physical, emotional, and spiritual self. It was during that time of self-reflection that I discovered a brand new path for my future. In a million years, I never would have thought that a small bottle of essential oil could have done so much, but it turns out that sometimes the smallest things are the most powerful. dōTERRA became a major catalyst in my decision to change paths personally *and* professionally, and I will be eternally grateful for that first exposure!

My intent in this particular article is not to expound on what essential oils have done for my health and wellness, although those experiences are numerous and profoundly important to me. Suffice to say, through the use of a number of holistic solutions—essential oils, food, stress management, and exercise—I boosted my immunity, supported healthy joint function, and got a grip on my stress and long-standing mood swings. On its own, this would have been huge, but it was only the beginning.

Beyond what essential oils did for my health was what the business of dōTERRA did for me personally and professionally. Yes, the business is financially rewarding, but it is much more than a paycheck to me. This business and the network marketing business model enabled me to take control of my life, my health, my schedule, and my income in a way that I never thought possible. I shifted my mindset about money and how I could harness the power of leverage to generate income. Throughout my professional career, I knew how to leverage the assets I had to make them go further—money and income are no different! I focused on building knowledge of holistic living and natural healing to gain insight into what people actually need to make their lives better. Most importantly, I got rid of the excuses I had been using for years to settle for less than I deserved.

Today, I work to live; I no longer live to work. Today, I know what my priorities are and I have arranged my life to accommodate them. Today, I am empowered, inspired, and excited about the path I'm on, where it is taking my family and me, and what is on the horizon. I am a human-being, no longer a human-doing.

I used to think I was defined by what I did. I was a Naval Officer, I was a management consultant, I was an entrepreneur, and I was a wife and mother. What I discovered through my journey with essential oils is that I am so much more than what I do; I am defined by who I am. I am a compassionate healer and someone who truly and passionately cares about the women I work with. Through my journey with dōTERRA, I learned to recognize my inherent introvert, accept it, but nonetheless open myself to the possibility of true fellowship and love from other amazing women who share my vision. I am a confident leader and someone who can inspire others to achieve their own dreams—no matter how out of reach they may seem. I am a wife and mother and entrepreneur and triathlete and woman and daughter and friend. I am all of these things but so much more than the sum of my parts.

I always wanted to live an inspired, exciting life full of possibility. What I now know is that my happiness lies in a life filled with purpose, love, and intention. The road less traveled, while sometimes filled with potholes and thorny bushes, leads to the most extraordinary destinations. I would never choose to trade those experiences for they are what makes life life—my life.

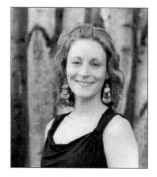

Merideth Cohrs is a business coach, speaker and the founder of Essential Oil Athlete. A graduate of the United States Naval Academy and the Institute for Integrative Nutrition, Merideth is an expert in leadership and mentoring, business and mindset coaching, and over 100 nutritional theories and practical lifestyle coaching applications. She is currently training to complete her first 70.3 Ironman triathlon and feels passionately about using physical exercise as a catalyst for life change. Merideth lives in Issaquah, Washington, with her husband, son, and two dogs.
Learn more: www.essentialoilathlete.com.

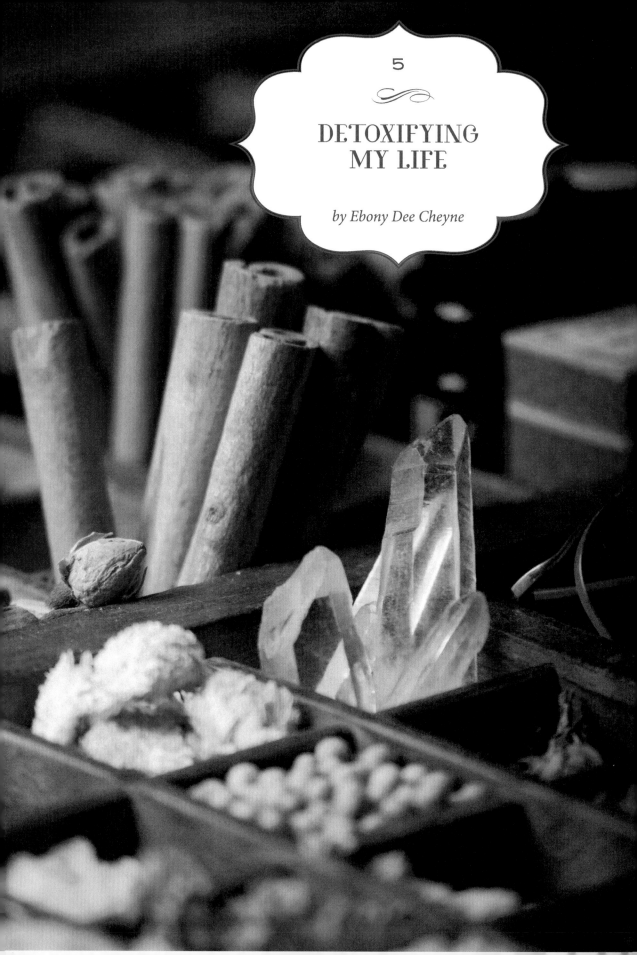

5

DETOXIFYING MY LIFE

by Ebony Dee Cheyne

The day after I graduated from art college, I went to live and work in the world of Hollywood's rich and famous. I worked with most of my favorite celebrities, artists, photographers, and musicians as a Fashion Stylist and Post-Production Specialist. Although it seemed as if I was living the dream, the lifestyle began to take its toll. I worked very hard, often with very stressful, demanding deadlines, and my health declined dramatically. On the outside I seemed fine, but on the inside I was dealing with a long list of increasingly debilitating health issues. My life was unraveling— there were no answers, and I was scared.

During this time, I moved to Paris to pursue my photography career and to seek a change in work/life balance. I started to educate myself slowly about how to take care of myself—I had a lot to learn! There is so much information and it was overwhelming to know what to believe. I knew that my priority had to be to change my whole lifestyle in order to regain and support my well-being. This catapulted the quest to support my body naturally and eventually led me to discovering dōTERRA essential oils.

When I discovered dōTERRA's products, I was astounded by how my body responded. I dove in, transforming and detoxifying my life in every area I could. I stopped using questionable chemicals to clean, on my skin, hair, teeth, to wash my clothes—all overnight. I started diffusing everywhere, taking supplements, and using single oils and blends that I absolutely adore.

Ironically, my lifestyle before my journey with dōTERRA *seemed* to be extremely exciting and glamorous despite all my difficulties. On the surface, I was living the dream by most people's standards—a lifestyle that many people believe will bring them happiness, wealth, and glamour. I was lucky enough to meet some of the most incredibly talented and influential people, earned well, led a pretty lavish lifestyle, and travelled the world. However, the most significant difficulty became apparent when I was unable to work and I had no income. If I missed a deadline, I would lose clients and my reputation along with my paychecks—plus, there was no sick pay for a freelancer/small business owner. In some cases, I had to be ready to drop everything at a moment's notice if I wanted the work. These factors led to a very unbalanced lifestyle.

Over time, my idea of glamour has changed dramatically. It does not include stressing myself out about finding the perfect outfit and jewels for celebrities that would keep the advertisers happy, or chaining myself to a computer for days making people look better than they could ever look naturally. Never knowing what my next month will look like financially is *not* glamorous. We have the technology to make almost *anything* look good these days, but what really matters is looking after the inside, first and foremost. Too often, we forget that.

Now I know that a truly glamorous lifestyle is being able to decline jobs that do not resonate, challenge, or make me happy and being able to work with people I respect. In any field, working with people who inspire each other every day to break new ground is so exciting. To work with those who genuinely want me to be my best self is a privilege.

It always bothered me that I never had the feeling I was helping to change the world in a positive way. But, like most people, I would push that feeling aside. I was helping the team or client create a vision and loved being a part of that process. But, in the bigger picture, there is nothing more rewarding than actually connecting with people at a very real level. I wanted a gut feeling of satisfaction, of doing something positive. I struggled with that for years.

DōTERRA has allowed me to shift focus to really make a difference on a much deeper level, and helping others love themselves from the inside out is my true passion. My experience has taught me that true beauty really comes from the inside. In a great photograph there is that inner sparkle of authentic self that shines through; you cannot make that up. I want everyone to have that sparkle.

I love that I can still collaborate with celebrity, fashion and music clients that I respect and admire. Gradually, however, my focus has been on how to make the inside beautiful. My own journey of health and has evolved to me choosing to share the best of what I have learned personally through this experience. Teaching other people I connect with in all areas of life about essential oils inevitably leads to embarking on a powerful discovery for us both, and it is an honor to be a part of that.

Having worked for many of the world's top brands, I am extremely difficult to impress with products. One of the reasons I chose dōTERRA for personal use was the quality—the industry-changing standards they go through to supply the very best and effective oils. A key part of this is their sustainable co-impact sourcing. The rare and incredible ethics of dōTERRA's core mission and that of everyone who is associated with the company have brought me to tears.

Typically, starting a successful business is only possible for those who can make large investments financially and have the ability to work full time—or more. There is a growing respect for network marketing for a reason. With a reputable company and amazing products, almost anyone can succeed with some determination. It is a profession I am very proud and grateful to be a part of, especially with the public support from Bill Gates, Tony Robbins, and Richard Branson, amongst many other very smart business mentors.

This is a choice for people who want to change their own lives, to change other people's lives, to do business fairly, come from a truly authentic place, and have no limits of possible financial freedom. The passion for the product naturally drives people to share, so it is all about making it accessible. The education dōTERRA provides is groundbreaking. To create a healer in every home is something I am very inspired by, as most of us know very little about our own bodies but complain when we have problems and seek a quick fix. In contrast, dōTERRA has taught me to love, respect, believe in, and truly know myself in many ways.

With my independent, entrepreneurial spirit, freedom of how to spend my time was always a great priority to me. My driving force and motivation for making career choices was always lifestyle. When I finally realized I still did not have freedom over my own time or my lifestyle and that my body was suffering, I knew something had to change and quickly. I chose to make the shift from very happy dōTERRA customer who was sharing the oils to a committed builder in the business. And that was the start of the true journey. I feel so lucky that I can have a great career centered on looking after myself properly. I never thought yoga classes, self-care appointments, and social events would become my job and that most of my training would be in personal growth. But becoming a leader in the world of dōTERRA has enabled huge personal growth physically, emotionally, professionally, and financially. Without even realizing it, most importantly, dōTERRA has supported me to become the leader of my own life. This journey has surprised me too many times to mention and continues to do so. Not only is my body in better shape than it has been for a very long time, but I am happier and supported in all ways. My life has been transformed.

If this business can work for me, it can work for anyone. Only a few years ago I was living a totally different lifestyle. If somebody had told me where I would be now, I would have never believed them. This shift doesn't mean losing ambition, or style, or personality. Quite the opposite! I can still work with major fashion (and other coveted) clients. However, I have achieved a life balance where my priority is to stay healthy and go to yoga and socialize with lovely, genuine people on a deeper level and spend time around my loved ones. How I run my life is now my choice. The only thing that competes with that satisfaction and of seeing people's health blossom is leading others to do the same.

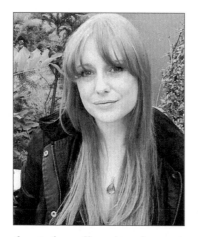

*Ebony Dee Cheyne, based in the UK, discovered dōTERRA whilst living as a fashion photographer in Paris, France. Her brand and website, Madame Bonheur, is named after the childhood character "Little Miss Happy." Oils, health, and happiness are the primary focus. Ebony is now combining her experience and skills to offer her worldwide team their own custom websites and photography, and will soon even offer retreats in Europe and beyond to help others teach about the oils, stylishly and effectively. Ebony's time freedom allowed her to train very closely with Hayley Hobson and many other top essential oil experts and health professionals in the USA and beyond, which enables her to be well equipped to train people in Europe and all over the world to do the same. Her motivation comes from seeing people smile and instantly feel great, often transforming in many ways with these oils, and the journey that evolves from that first experience. **Learn more: www.madamebonheur.com.***

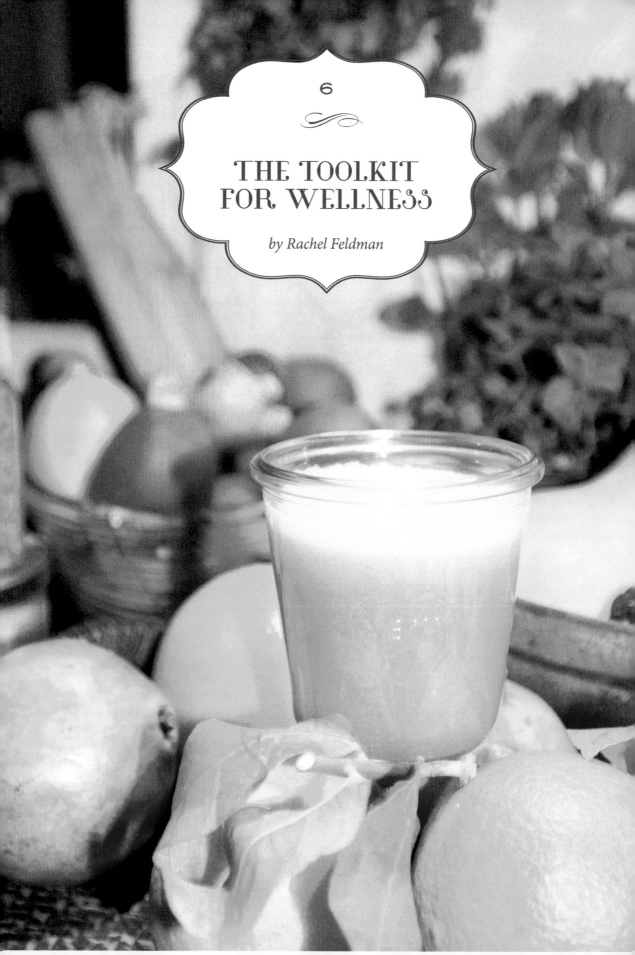

6

THE TOOLKIT FOR WELLNESS

by Rachel Feldman

AS A HEALTH COACH AND DETOX SPECIALIST, PEOPLE OFTEN ASSUME THAT I HAVE ALWAYS BEEN THE PICTURE OF PERFECT HEALTH. I WISH I COULD TELL YOU THAT MY LIFE HAS BEEN FREE OF HEALTH CHALLENGES, BUT THAT'S NOT THE CASE.

I was a very active kid and swam competitively throughout my childhood and teens. But something was off. I suffered from allergies, hormonal imbalances, and stomach issues. At age fourteen, I developed my first ulcer, which eventually turned into ulcerative colitis, considered an autoimmune disease. I developed asthma at age eighteen, which landed me in the hospital monthly and even on life support multiple times.

I remember saying to my Mom at one point in my twenties, "I think I'm dying." The shock on her face was enough to shatter my heart. Here I was—young, thriving professionally as a commercial real estate broker, and I looked healthy. But I had been battling these issues for the bulk of my life and didn't seem to be getting any better.

I was told, "You have toxicity, pathogens, adrenal fatigue, and hormonal imbalances and your digestive system is very inflamed." I went from doctor to doctor, each time hopeful for a magical plan or protocol, but nobody could tell me why my tests were abnormal or what to do to feel better.

I finally came to the realization that my journey to Wellsville had to start with me. Intuitively, I knew there was another way, and I set out to find it. That day I took the first step on the path that made me who I am today: a mom, health coach, detox specialist, and the proud business owner of Rachel's Wellness.

I read every book I could get my hands on and spent hours on the Internet researching about my health. I learned about foods that could restore my gut and supplements and tinctures that would support my health. I started exploring alternative therapies—acupuncture and Chinese medicine, among others.

One of the natural solutions I learned about was essential oils. Back then, fifteen years ago, they were not as popular as they are today. But luckily for me, my favorite little health food store in Philadelphia carried them.

My hormonal issues took some time to turn around. It had gotten to the point where doctors told me I would never get pregnant. Devastated by that news, I had a session with an energy worker who told me she was going to clear my cells. She added essential oils to some coconut oil and massaged them into my body and near my uterus. She told me the prolactin levels would lessen, and I would be ready to conceive.

I got pregnant on my honeymoon a month later! I am not claiming this would work for everyone, but I do know this: Essential oils penetrate the cell on a physical and emotional level, releasing blockages. You can bet your bottom dollar I sent birth announcements to the doctors who said I would never conceive!

I was so grateful for the information and practitioners who had helped me in my wellness journey that I couldn't in good faith not share it with others. I made a decision to leave my job to deepen my knowledge of health at the Institute of Integrative Nutrition.

When I graduated and began working with clients as a health coach, I observed the powerful impact detoxing and changing the diet could have on their well-being. But I was still seeing some of my clients suffer health problems on a deeper cellular level. Food is a big part of the equation, but I learned that sometimes even the cleanest eaters still face health challenges. We live in a world polluted with toxins, emotional and physical. So I continued to research how I could further support my clients to be their healthiest selves.

Having this toolkit in my house has been nothing short of life changing. Every day I put On Guard®, Balance™, Lemon, and Peppermint on the soles of my kids' feet for immune support, great sleep, and healthy cleansing.

I use essential oils like Frankincense, On Guard, Melaleuca, InTune®, Balance, and Elevation myself every day, and when I don't, I feel off. I have diffusers in every room of my house. I add citrus oils such as Lemon, Grapefruit, and Orange to my water. I use Slim & Sassy® for my metabolism. I am empowered when it comes to my health and well-being.

I am also empowered in my business. Never in my wildest dreams did I think I would help other health warriors, coaches, moms or friends to learn about essentials oils and then make money. Every month I get a check in the mail, I laugh because I am getting paid for doing something I love, which is sharing the beauty of essential oils and how they work.

Not only did we get empowered emotionally and physically but we got empowered financially. I am saving these checks for college tuition.

Thanks to detoxing regularly and supporting my body with a natural approach, I am thriving and so is my family. I believe that being healthy and vibrant is the birthright of each and every one of us, and I am dedicated to supporting that birthright through my work. I believe it is our birthright to love what we do. I make a healthy income in my health coaching practice and with essential oils. Pretty awesome, right? I simply share what I do in my life.

I couldn't be happier doing what I do—teaching busy people how to detox and eat cleanly and how to support their health with the highest-quality essential oils. I feel privileged to have found my path to serve. My children tell people,

"Mommy helps people to get better." I didn't start with the intention to build a business with essential oils. I was just looking for a solution for my family and for the clients I thought could benefit from the oils. But I got so passionate about these products when I started to see my family and my clients thrive, wellness professionals began to ask me more about them, and organically a business was born.

It feels great to be able to stand behind a product that you know to be of the highest quality—and to help others do the same. Being able to empower my team to share their passion for the power of essential oils to supplement their income or—be their primary income—has been truly inspiring. I have helped wellness professionals, moms, nurses, and other like-minded people follow their dreams and become financially independent.

I'm not sure there are many jobs out there where you get to teach people about powerful and natural ways to take charge of their health and get paid for it. I look forward to my checks from dōTERRA, but, more importantly, I look forward to coaching my team to help change this world, one oil at a time!

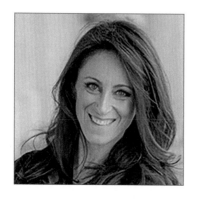

Rachel Feldman is a health coach, wellness momma, and a detox specialist. Rachel graduated from the Institute for Integrative Nutrition in New York City, Wild Rose Natural College of Healing, and the International School of Detoxification and Natalia Rose Advanced Detox Certification Training. She is also certified by the American Association of Drugless Practitioners and has obtained additional Continuing Education Units from Purchase College, State University of New York. Her approach to health focuses not only on the foods you put into your mouth but also incorporates the elements of the body, mind, and soul. She is also a biz coach for health-focused solopreneurs, helping you create more, get your work out there strategically, and start raking in the cash you deserve. She has a successful health coaching practice. She uses a proven system in her thriving practice—these are the tools she sells to health coaches. She does not just write the programs, she uses them, too! Ready to empower your business? Learn more: www.rachelswellness.com; www.detox.rachelswellness.com.

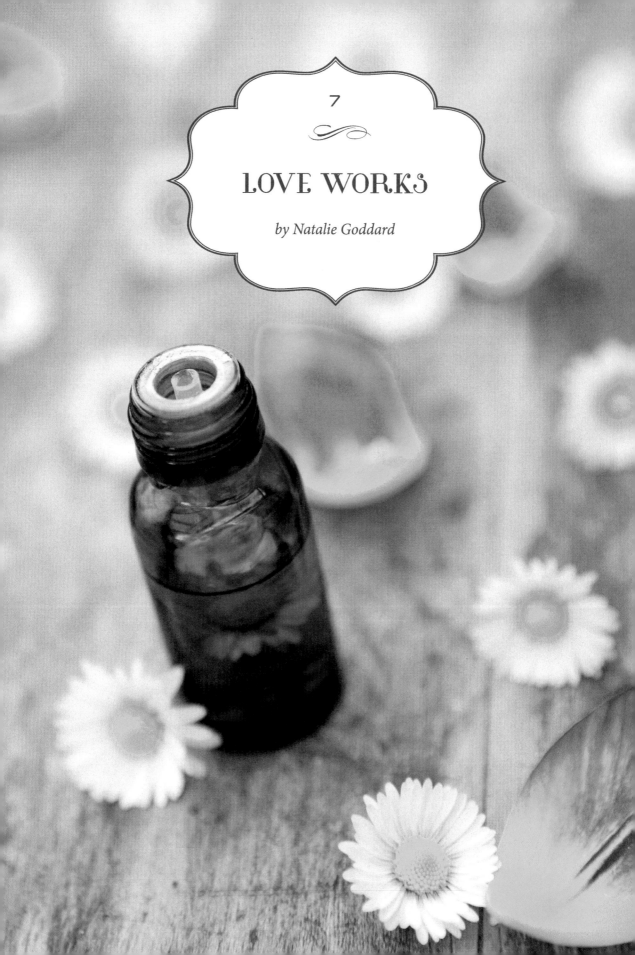

7

LOVE WORKS

by Natalie Goddard

"Something amazing happens when we surrender and just love. We melt into another world, a realm of power already within us."

—Marianne Williamson

I GREW UP IN A SMALL TOWN. MY DAD RAISED US ON A CATTLE RANCH WHERE I WAS TAUGHT THAT LIFE IS A STRUGGLE. THERE WERE SCARCE RESOURCES IN THIS DOG-EAT-DOG WORLD, SO IT WAS EVERY MAN FOR HIMSELF, AND I LEARNED SUCCESS COMES TO THOSE WHO HELP THEMSELVES.

My mom died when I was 19, and this drastically changed my world. She meant everything to me, and with her gone, I quickly felt like my life was in shambles.

I turned to God for answers and did mission work. I went to school and did all kinds of volunteer work in an effort to find myself. I learned some lessons along the way, but still hoped for the ache in my heart to end.

After the birth of our second child, my loneliness grew and I found myself in full-blown depression. I still remember the day my hope was born again. Andy had purchased me a massage with a woman who used essential oils with music and massage. And it made me feel hopeful. I came home with essential oils and began to swipe them on my husband and our children. I felt a love of life coming back as my heart began to be healed by the oils.

On a summer afternoon in 2008, I was driving down the road with my children. I saw a woman feeding horses by the road with her children. I had the impression, "Stop and talk to that woman." I ignored it at first. "I'm not a stalker," I thought. Again, the impression came to turn the car around and talk to her. So I did.

She introduced herself and we spoke for a while and exchanged contact information. She emailed me a few weeks later and invited me to an introductory class on dōTERRA essential oils. I attended only after she persisted several times.

When I attended the class, they claimed to have the purest essential oils on planet earth. I rolled my eyes and thought, "I've heard that before." Then they passed the Peppermint oil around the class and I was blown away. "How could anything else I've experienced before have even be called peppermint?" I asked.

Then they passed the Frankincense to me. Before I even opened it, I could feel a difference. There seemed to be a vibration to it that was tangible. I opened the bottle, and I actually started to cry. I had a very clear impression enter my mind saying: "Pay attention."

Teresa Harding told me about the opportunity to be in the Founder's Club. I was intrigued, but I couldn't imagine myself being successful. I had major blocks about network marketing. As a mom of four, I felt like others could do this and be successful, but not me. I had kids, a full life, and since I was totally committed to my family, I didn't want anything taking away from our time together.

One day, as I was driving, I asked God what He had in store for me. I told Him I wanted to be successful in dōTERRA but I had some blocks. The clear impression I got was that He wanted me to be successful, but if I chose out, He would give it to someone else. He gave the classic takeaway and I worked to pull me in.

Since then, we've received impressions to share the oils with many people in our lives. Following those impressions and seeing the oils and the business bless lives has been one of the most rewarding experiences of our lives.

Sharing dōTERRA has been the single greatest learning experience I've had. What I've learned is almost exactly the opposite of what I learned growing up on the ranch. Here's how I would sum it all up in two words: Love works. It's not greed that works, or recognition, or fame. *Love* is the key to influence, leadership, and success.

There were times when I was building dōTERRA that I was driven by pride. Sometimes, I wanted recognition. Sometimes I wanted to prove I was better than another builder. But one of my mentors, Tiffany Peterson, taught me to *serve more to sell more. I* found that when I came from a place of service and a desire to serve the person I was with, I had more success *and* more fun. If I focus on me, I get weak results. But if I forget myself in service, I can be totally present and change their life.

It's amazing how humbling it can be to build a dōTERRA business. It seems to expose all of my weaknesses! But when the student is ready, a teacher always appears.

I remember one time I stood in front of a room of 100 women to teach them about dōTERRA. I was so nervous I almost threw up! And I didn't have any enrollments from my presentation! I knew something needed to change if I was going to be successful.

Right after that nerve-wracking presentation, I read a quote by Byron Katie (I highly recommend her book, *Loving What Is*). She said, "When I walk into a room, I know that everyone in it loves me. I just don't expect them to realize it yet."

At first I thought she was so pretentious! But after attending two of her live seminars, I realized that she is so grounded that she only holds a space for love in her life. At that point I had a decision to make: What will I let run my show?

I've learned that the purpose of my life is really simple: to love and be loved. At my core, I'm a little girl who loves to be loved and needs to be needed.

Life is just a cycle of giving and receiving love. In this cycle, you get to set the pace. If you want to receive more love, give more away.

It's been super useful for me to think of my dōTERRA genealogy as a tree of love. The company and your upline are your roots, you are the trunk, and your downline is your branches. The love flows from the owners and from your upline. If you want the tree to be healthy, would you ever think of cutting the tree at the base (excluding or bad-talking your upline)? Think how much it hurts you *and* your team if you leave your upline out of your events or team calls.

Every great story is a story of love.
Love believes.
Love gives and shares—whether it be samples or your focus when you are with someone.
Love remembers—have a plan or a system for follow-up so they know you care.
Love tries again.
Love never gives up.
Love leads.
Love listens.
Love follows.
Love creates value.
Love serves.

Now I enjoy a sweet life with my amazing companion and seven unique children. We have a team of more than 430,000 people around the world whom we love and pray for and partner with. I celebrate the gift of love and life. I love the way I am stretched to love more as I build dōTERRA. I honor you for sharing this journey and choosing love.

If you ever feel alone, discouraged, or disappointed, try love. It works. Try soaking it in. Try passing it on.

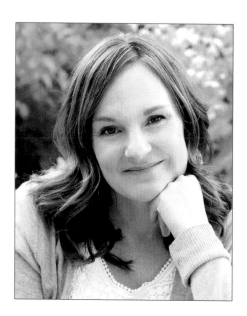

Natalie Goddard *is passionate about empowering mommas to find real answers within. She loves watching dōTERRA change lives! She is a devoted wife and mother, dōTERRA Double Diamond, Co-Creator of Share Success, a Holistic Health Coach, and a Marriage and Family Life Educator. She thrives on working hard creating content and sharing it, playing hard in nature with her seven amazing children, and following her intuition to make a difference one on one or through charity.* **Learn more: www.naturalsolutionsrevolution.com.**

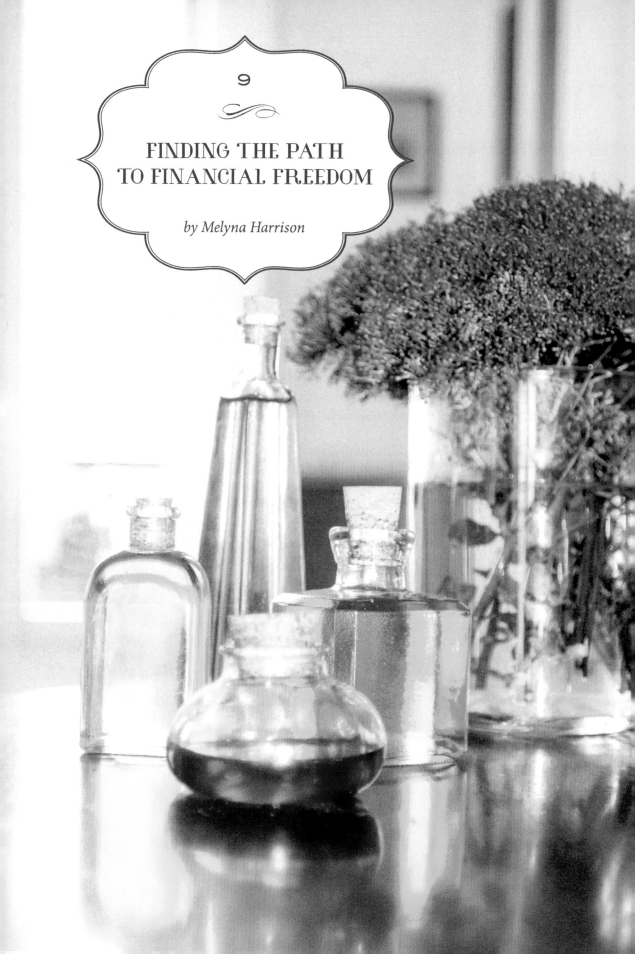

9

FINDING THE PATH TO FINANCIAL FREEDOM

by Melyna Harrison

I WAS FORTUNATE TO BE RAISED IN A VERY NATURAL HOME. EVERY MEAL WAS MADE AT HOME FROM SCRATCH, USING ONLY WHOLE-FOOD INGREDIENTS AND NEVER INCLUDING ANY REFINED SUGARS. BUT THERE WERE GAPS. AS A MASSAGE THERAPIST, I KNEW A LITTLE ABOUT ESSENTIAL OILS AND THEIR CALMING ABILITIES. BUT ONCE I UNDERSTOOD HOW POWERFUL ESSENTIAL OILS ARE WHEN SOURCED APPROPRIATELY, I JUST HAD TO SHARE THEM WITH OTHERS.

In the beginning, I wasn't concerned with bringing in an income so much as I wanted to share something I had known about sooner. My husband John had an extremely successful business. But then—he didn't. Overnight, he lost the company and all our savings. Before long, we lost our home and our cars. We were newly pregnant with our third child. We had two business partners who we considered family, and they were in the exact same situation, both families also pregnant with their third baby. It almost seemed like a bad dream that we were going to wake up from at any minute.

Because I had been consistently sharing dōTERRA with others for about a year, I had created an income of about $1,500 per month. But that wasn't enough to support our family! Where were we going to live? How were we going to feed our family? How were we going to pay our health insurance? How were we going to support yet another child? We knew we had to take control of the situation and get our lives back. We moved in with my mom. John got two jobs, and I started to see dōTERRA for what it really could do for my family. It was hard to spend a lot of time on it with my husband always gone and two young kids at home with me, not to mention a belly that kept growing. I would wake up early and get to work. I would put a movie on for my daughter while my son napped, and I would work. After bedtime I would stay up late and work.

There were definitely some sacrifices made, but I was grateful that I was the one who got to choose which sacrifices to make so that I could fit the work around my busy life as a mother. I remember the day my daughter started kindergarten. I had committed to be at an event in Vegas because I really needed to grow my business. It was a choice that I knew I had to make, and my mom took pictures for me, but I cried all the way there. Because we had moved to another state, I had to drive six hours back to Nevada for all my prenatal doctor's visits. I couldn't change insurance since I was already pregnant, and I couldn't afford to pay the out-of-network costs to have a baby. I would have my mom watch my kids while I drove the 12-hour round trip. Each time I traveled I would do a couple events so that I could get my gas reimbursed through dōTERRA's Diamond Club program, and so I could continue to grow my team.

After the baby was born, it was harder to balance things, but we kept working and hit the rank of Platinum that month. A year after the financial reset button was pushed, I had tripled my income, so I was able to convince John to come home so we could really focus on dōTERRA and I could participate in Diamond Club once more. This was a very scary decision because we still weren't really able to support a family *and* a business while I traveled and sponsored a handful of other team members in Diamond Club as well. We knew we had to hit that next level if we were going to make it. With baby in tow, I hit the road, and a few months later we became dōTERRA Diamonds, then Blue Diamonds, then Presidential Diamonds.

As I look back on our path to financial freedom, it wasn't always pretty. There were times I was so exhausted I could hardly think. My children didn't get as much attention as I wanted to give them. They ate more pizza dinners and watched more television than I care to admit, and at times I felt like I was failing as a mother. But I loved the mission of empowerment that I was on, and I knew the sacrifices we were making were worthwhile. I tried to make up for my absence by applying oils nightly with lots of hugs and kisses. Little by little we were able to create the life we wanted.

While pregnant with our fourth child last summer, we decided to step back a little from building and move our family to Mexico for three months so we could spend some quality time making memories together. The awesome thing is that our business still continued to grow! I was also able to outsource a lot of my responsibilities so I could be more effective and focus on specific things in my life. We hired help to clean my house and cook a couple times a week. We hired a personal assistant to handle a big portion of our business, which gave us freedom to grow more. We hired a nanny to come four mornings a week to be with the kids while we worked, so they were actively engaged instead of in front of the TV. And in the process we are providing good jobs for others.

We don't worry anymore about how we are going to pay the bills. I made the leap of faith into myself and was able to create a life with endless possibilities. I get to work with my best friend, and my children not only have a mother at home with them but they get a full time daddy at home as well. We have financial freedom and know that we could stop working today and be just fine. But every time I think about stopping I think back to that first experience I had applying oils on my baby. I think of all the other mothers out there who feel that same helpless feeling I felt as they hold their child in their arms wishing they could do more. I want to empower them so they have options!

I think back to the times when we had to stretch every penny and still came up short each month. I know I have team members who still feel that way and wish they could hire some help. I want to empower them so that they have options! I think of the times that my husband was bringing home a great income but was stressed and gone so much of the time. I was lonely, and he only saw his kids an hour or two each night, and even then he was so exhausted that he just wanted to relax instead of play with them like he does now. I think about the families all over the world who feel the same way. They are living their jobs and trying desperately to fit their life in around their work instead of the other way around. I want to empower them so that they have options. And that is what is so rewarding for me— the ripple effect of what we have created.

We only have one life. We need to live it to the fullest of our capacity, and with financial freedom and time freedom, everything else falls into place.

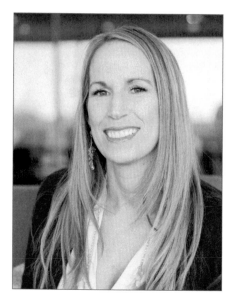

Melyna Harrison is a wife and mother of four young children. With a background in massage therapy, essential oils came naturally for her. Originally when she joined dōTERRA it was simply because she fell in love with the wonderful products and her husband considered this a fun "hobby" for her. Because of her natural understanding of the business and her passion for educating others, she found herself replacing her husband's income after two years. Now, Melyna and her husband John work together from home leading an amazing team of people as Presidential Diamonds. **Learn more: www.mydoterra.com/eopro; essentialoilpro@gmail.com.**

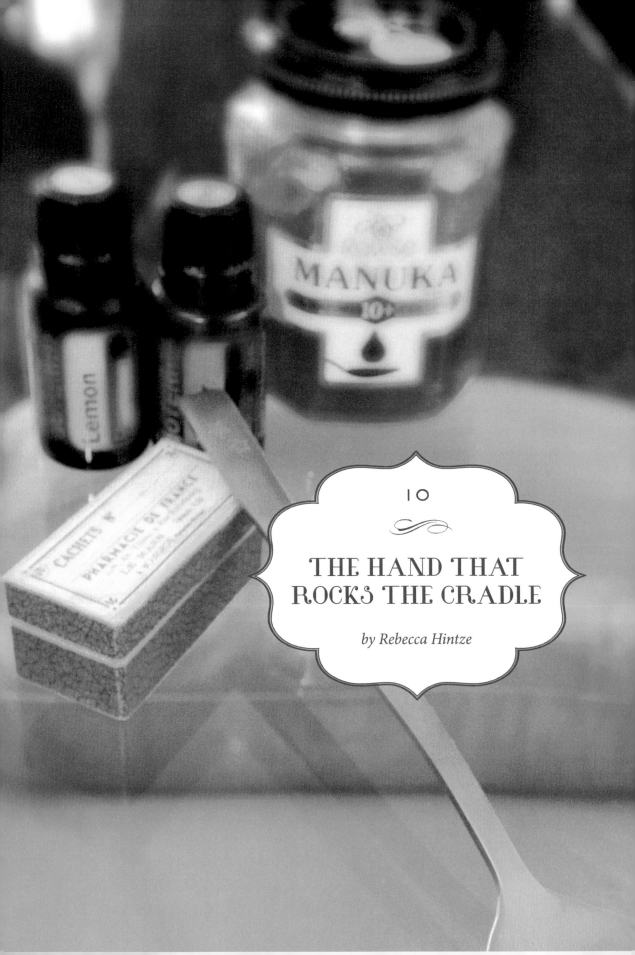

10

❧

THE HAND THAT ROCKS THE CRADLE

by Rebecca Hintze

I LOVE THE WILLIAM ROSS WALLACE QUOTE "THE HAND THAT ROCKS THE CRADLE IS THE HAND THAT RULES THE WORLD!" IT'S TRUE.

When I compiled data for one of my books, *Healing Your Family History*, I calculated how many people descend from a couple who marry and have three children, with the pattern of marrying and bearing three children continuing for a dozen generations. The total descending from the original couple over time was in the millions—3,188,643, to be exact. Often, we think if we want to change the world that we need to leave our homes and work in some profound position that leads to notoriety and worldly praise. The truth is, there's no more important work than the efforts put forth within our homes, with our spouse or partner, and with our children.

My journey with essential oils began in 2008. A friend called me on several occasions and insisted I purchase some. Not only was I not very interested in essential oils, I definitely was not interested in buying anything from a network marketing company. However, I love my friend and I trusted her instincts. So, I caved—one of the best decisions I've ever made. I opened a wholesale account with what would become a billion-dollar company and the largest supplier of essential oils in the world: dōTERRA.

As soon as my initial order arrived, I began using and loving essential oils daily. In fact, within two weeks, nearly every bottle I ordered was empty. What was happening? My family was falling in love with essential oils! It didn't take long before I became an essential oil junky, packing these products everywhere—family picnics, long car rides, even tubing down the nearby Shenandoah River—I didn't want to go anywhere without them. And I wasn't alone. My children and husband shared the same passion. We were smitten with the products and the company. We began to wonder what our lives would be without them.

Why? Good question! After years of looking into natural ways to uplift mood and support healthy immunity and overall wellness, I had finally found my answer. I wanted to tell everyone: "There are natural solutions to support optimal well-being and they actually work!"

To my surprise, my "roof-top shouting" self handed me an unexpected surprise—a fast-growing network marketing business. After all, telling everyone about essential oils and powerful nutritional products meant I had to tell people where to buy them, and, well, the rest is history. Today, we—my husband and I—are among the top distributors of a billion-dollar direct sales company. This unexpected opportunity left my husband retiring from his Vice President executive status position at a publicly traded U.S. company just four years after that first box of oils arrived on our porch.

So what does all of this have to do with family? After all, that's where this conversation began.

After working more than twenty years in the field of mental health, I've witnessed countless lives damaged from destructive behaviors, limiting beliefs, unhappiness, and poor health. I've studied nutrition and brain chemistry, as well as patterns of health among families, and I've written books about happiness, health, and improving mood. Truly, what affects one, impacts others. We are connected in this large universe—and we are most certainly connected as families, both genetically and emotionally. If individuals have the power to change the world over time (remember that large figure I started with?), the more we support powerful personal change, the better the future of our world (assuming those we support procreate and pass along a healthier message to future generations).

Here's the answer to that question: Essential oils and healthy nutrition are both instrumental in improving mood and managing healthy cellular communication, ultimately supporting the recovery of both the individual and the family over time. In short, these simple solutions Mother Nature provides may be enhancing mood, improving intuition, spawning improved social and interpersonal connections, and generally uplifting the outlook of those who use them.

If this is the case, the impact of using these simple and inexpensive tools may have far greater reaching affects on our world than the simple support many find when they reach to a bottle of Lavender or Orange to feel peace and calm, or they take a supplement to enhance their health. Yes, essential oils and nutritional support changed my life and my family's life, but that's a small number of people (seven, to be exact) compared to the support these compounds may provide to my posterity over time (remember, we're talking millions). Some may assume I'm suggesting that my kids will share essential oils and supplements with their kids and the physical taking of these products would provide that outcome. That's not what I'm suggesting—though I do hope that familial sharing and good health habits continue on beyond my life. What I'm suggesting is that as individuals perhaps our own personal healing (because we've used essential oils and nutrition to support us) may leave us better connected as human beings, better able to communicate effectively with our loved ones and to bond with infants, and more equipped to provide loving and healthy communication in our homes. If this happens, the fruits of these efforts are beyond what we realize.

According to well-recognized psychologists John Bowby (from the UK) and Mary Ainsworth (from the U.S.), the relationship between a mother and her child sets the precedent for all future relationships and communication techniques that child will experience in the future. Our world is built on relationships and communication—starting at home with families and ultimately reaching to extend worldwide. Back to my point, "The hand that rocks the cradle is the hand that rules the world." Any support we provide primary care-givers and enhance the ability of families to grow in loving, healthy, connected ways will go a long way in changing the world.

Yes, essential oils work! They help families feel better physically and emotionally. Yes, nutrition is essential for our emotional and physical well-being; our brains and bodies need nutrition to function properly. Citrus essential oils support healthy brain function in the sense that they are natural mood up-lifters, and many essential oils support a healthy nervous system. All these things are documented in science today. And as such, they are helpful for families to know about today—thus, the "roof-top shouting" that's going on! But the long-term effects of this global change toward natural solutions for health care may be even more powerful down the road—if mothers and fathers use these tools to better the relationships they have with their children, seek to improve mood, and desire to grow together in unshakeable family bonds that ultimately leave families passing along constructive patterns, healthy belief systems, and long-lasting happiness. This is my wish, and my mission—to support the healing of families worldwide.

When I reluctantly enrolled as a dōTERRA Wellness Advocate, I had no idea that this experience would be a greater vehicle to help facilitate global change than writing books and providing counseling to families—the path I had been taking. I had no idea the blessings these products would provide for my children, and now my grandchildren. As a mental health professional, I wanted to change the world, and now I believe I've been given another tool that just might allow me to do just that!

A heart-felt thanks to the owners of my essential oil company for offering me such a gift—the gift of the earth.

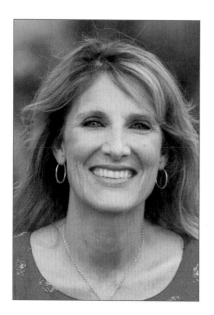

Rebecca Hintze, M.Sc., is a family issues expert and bestselling author of Healing Your Family History, Living Healthy and Happily Ever After, *and* Essentially Happy. *She has worked for more than two decades in the mental health field. Rebecca specializes in helping individuals break free of destructive patterns. She holds a bachelor's degree from Brigham Young University and an M.S. in Psychology from the University of East London. Rebecca is a former broadcast journalist and has appeared on national and international media, both as a journalist and as an expert guest educating on mental health issues. Rebecca and her husband, Shane, have been married for more than twenty-seven years. They have four grown children and two grandsons.* **Learn more: www.rebeccahintze.com.**

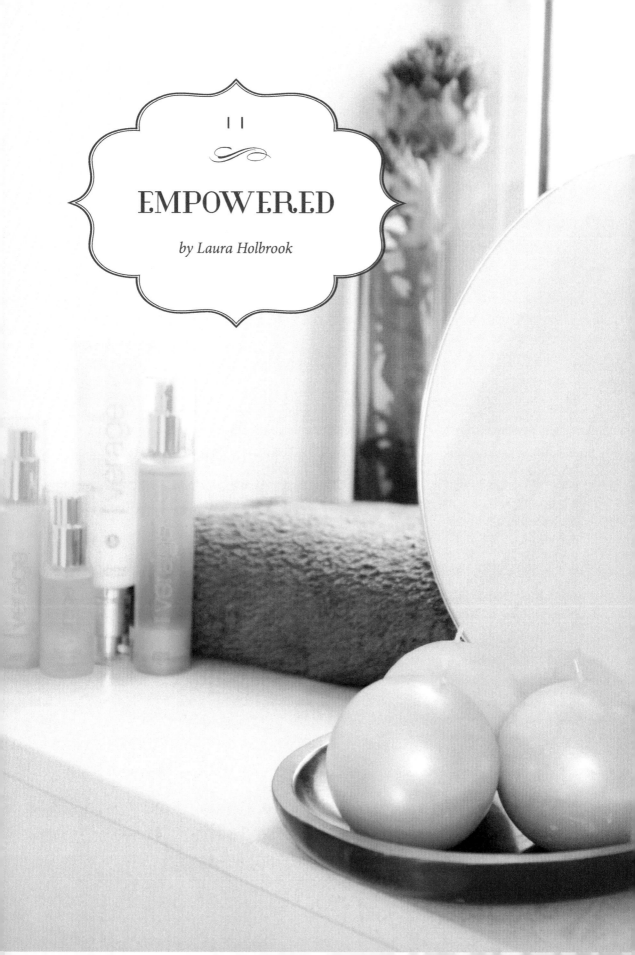

EMPOWERED

by Laura Holbrook

At fourteen, I made and sold T-shirts to friends and family. At fifteen, I began working as a contract seamstress. I was hardworking but not all that employable, because after working a job for a couple months I would start daydreaming about owning my business. I looked forward to someday being a mother and having the flexibility to raise my children at home.

At the same time, I had a fear of being left alone and not being able to provide. I had the belief that a man would provide the overall stability financially. I took that belief into adulthood. It was this battle in my own head: I want to be successful, but could I really do it? Could I make something significant?

By the time I was twenty-two, I had met and married my husband Wade. As we started a family, he enrolled in college. Ten years later, he had a master's degree and five daughters (and would eventually have a son as well). Through it all, I continued to sew, even starting an online mom and baby store. But I was making only a small profit, not leveraging my time, which was quite limited. I still had dreams of something better!

Wade is an entrepreneurial thinker too. After he graduated, he worked in the field of drug and alcohol treatment, and he saw a need for a transitional living place after people left rehab. We took a huge leap of faith as he quit his job and, together, we opened a Sober Living facility together. I taught yoga, nutrition, and life skill classes. He ran administrative, marketing, and public relations functions. I remember asking Wade how long before he thought we would be profitable and make $10,000 a month—the magic number I had for success!—and he speculated maybe five years.

As it turns out, we didn't have five years. As we attracted more clients, residents in that upper-end neighborhood pressured the city to change the client capacity ordinance so that we no longer could operate our facility. We were put out of business overnight, and our investment vanished!

From those depths of financial despair ten years ago, I was introduced to network marketing. I began to see the possibility of the networking message—that I could be with my family and earn money sharing their products. I liked the product and thought, why not? This could be something!

I heard someone say, "Would you rather be ignorance on fire or knowledge on ice?" And I became ignorance on fire! I began sharing and actually earned some money.

Although I was taking action and moving forward, I still had the nagging fear that I wasn't good enough somehow. I was terrified of sounding dumb, especially speaking in front of people. My mentor at the time told me that it was okay if I stumbled on my words. It was a good thing if the people I spoke in front of saw me as "human" and that they wouldn't bite me. That made me laugh and loosened me up a bit. I knew that I had to conquer this fear and stop doubting myself.

A big a-ha moment for me was when I was introduced to movie "The Secret" and recognized the part I played in limiting myself. I knew that this wall must come down.

The first time I presented, I was terrified. I faked confidence big time! The second time I spoke was at a luncheon and several top leaders attended and also brought people. I faked confidence in front of thirty people!

As I continued to just do it despite how I felt about myself, an awesome thing happened… I actually became confident. I had so many opportunities to grow (or fake it till I made it!). I even made a company-wide tool—a DVD that helped people create duplication in their teams. Did I have fears about doing it? Yes! I had cold hands and butterflies that day we filmed. Was it successful? Yes! Did people know I was nervous and felt bottled up? Probably not. I knew I must conquer my fears or they would forever hold me back. This led to me doing several short video clips and being featured in company literature.

Our business grew. In fact, the first year we hit top-ten income earners! Life was abundant and good. Then, in 2008, the economy collapsed and our check began to rapidly decline. The product we represented was one-dimensional and more of a commodity than a necessity. And so people began to turn off their auto-shipments. I began to really see how important it was to have experienced leadership in an economic change or crisis, and we didn't have that. I felt discouraged.

Looking back, that first networking experience prepared me for the blessings of dōTERRA. I learned what to look for in a company: a stable compensation plan, experienced leaders and owners, a multi-dimensional product (that is, something for everyone), and a clear company vision. And then I found dōTERRA. Wade and I were both completely impressed with the depth of experience the owners had. The culture was unlike anything we had ever experienced. "Compensation built like a rock" is what David Stirling told me. How true this was! This is what we were looking for—stability!

After researching the company, we jumped in with both feet. We were in! Making the move to build an essential oil business was the best decision we made.

I remember the day of our business launch. I was so nervous because I knew nothing about essential oils. I had only had a few experiences with them. I knew, however, because of my experiences so far that I could share what little I did know. I was beginning to feel like an empowered mom with these amazing oils.

At our launch we had about fifty people in attendance (and that included my large family). We hit Gold our first month. At the end of the fifth month, we achieved Diamond. We worked the business as if every day was a week. We had one-on-one appointments, business lunches, and daily classes, and traveled to areas where our team was beginning to grow. We nourished it one day at a time, one person at a time, one class at a time.

If I were to choose one word that would describe how I feel about being a business woman, it would be *empowered*. I am empowered as a mom of six kids to have these oils at my fingertips! I am empowered as a woman to have this wonderful business opportunity! It took me only two weeks to understand why my dōTERRA would be a billion-dollar company one day. Today, it *is* a billion-dollar company and we are just getting started! I will never be without them. They have saved us so much money. This is precisely why this business is recession-proof. It becomes a necessity, and that makes for a very powerful and long-lasting business.

The oils are a big part of our daily health and wealth. Our children know a good thing. We have every oil in our kitchen accessible to them. They know what works, and they know how to use them. I occasionally get texts from our kids asking me to bring them specific oils as their friends need them too.

My husband and I are now at the rank of Blue Diamond and we have more than 35,000 people in our organization. It has been an amazing—and uncomfortable—journey. I have mastered doing webinars while breastfeeding, three-way calls while changing dirty diapers, and teaching classes while having extreme morning sickness while pregnant with my little boy. I've planned many classes when no one shows up. Many people say no. But over time, they tend to come back with a yes.

If you want to grow this business, you have to be willing to get out of your comfort zone on a regular basis. This allows personal growth. And with that growth, comes a bigger paycheck. To get different results than you are currently getting, you have to do things differently today.

Consistent, small changes every day lead to big results. If I hadn't gotten out of my comfort zone ten years ago, I don't believe I would own the rank of Blue Diamond today. I employed the "fake it till you make it" with my public speaking. And I *did* make it. And if I did, why can't you? Every decision leads to the next opportunity. Personal growth never stops.

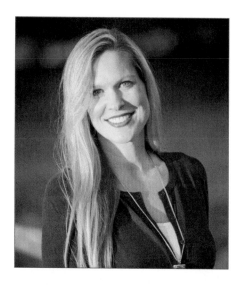

Laura Holbrook grew up in a big family—with four sisters and two brothers—and now she's raising a big family, with five daughters and a son. She is passionate about helping her daughters—and women, more generally—discover their potential and inner strength to do, be, and achieve their dreams. Laura is a nutritional advisor, certified personal fitness trainer, and certified yoga teacher with a DVD called "Essential Yoga" available in stores. Laura has been featured in SUCCESS *from* Home *magazine,* dōTERRA *Essential Leadership magazine, and* Networking Times *magazine. At their home in Utah, the Holbrooks enjoy fresh eggs from their chickens, honey from their bees, and produce year-round in their underground greenhouse.* **Learn more:** *laura@holbrook.org; facebook.com/laura.holbrook.*

THOUGHTS ON
LEADERSHIP

by Laura Holbrook

- **Plan your week ahead.** I have specific days when I do coaching calls. I do training every Tuesday with our weekly Booster call. I keep track of who I send samples to and when I follow up. By having a schedule, I keep myself as organized as possible—even with six kids! If I fail to plan, I plan to fail.

- **Keep it simple,** because however you share and teach about the products and the business, others will think that is what they need to do to build and share! If you make it complicated—like, discussing the detailed profile of Frankincense—people will feel that they could never do what you do. Keep presentations at a fifth-grade comprehension level.

- **Keep classes short,** no longer than 40 minutes. Even if the class is amazing, people will hesitate to come again if it's too long because of the time commitment.

- **At the end of each class, ask two key questions.** I call these the "million dollar questions." Sit one-on-one with the person and ask, "What did you like best?" This is open-ended and positive. We have two ears and one mouth. Use that! We ask and we listen. If we are doing most of the talking, we will not find out what the person's hot button is—that is, what interests them. It may feel unnatural to ask this, but trust me, it works! The next million-dollar question is, "Are you interested in learning how to get free products every month?" I have had no one tell me no. You then go on to explain the LRP program.

- When teaching a class or sharing the oils one-on-one, **always use a tool.** I like to use tear pads. By using a tool, you create duplication. I read from the tear sheet in front of me as I teach about the oils. Sure, I can do it without it, but I want to create duplication. I want people to know that they can do what I do! The last thing you want is someone complicating it and becoming confused. A confused mind always says no.

- **Make everything about them.** This is about your friend getting the best oils and getting the best discounts (wholesale account) and the most for free (LRP). Never make sharing the oils about you building your business or power of three. When you put others' needs first, your needs will be filled. Your business will grow.

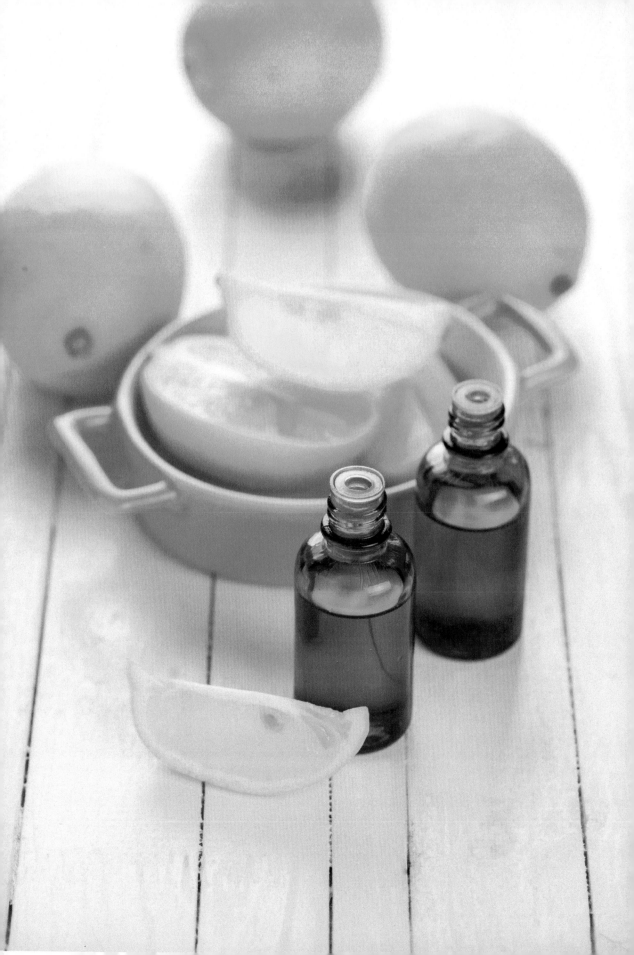

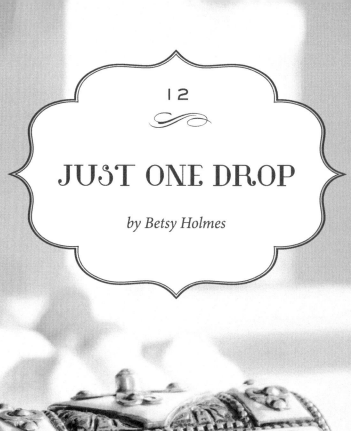

12

JUST ONE DROP

by Betsy Holmes

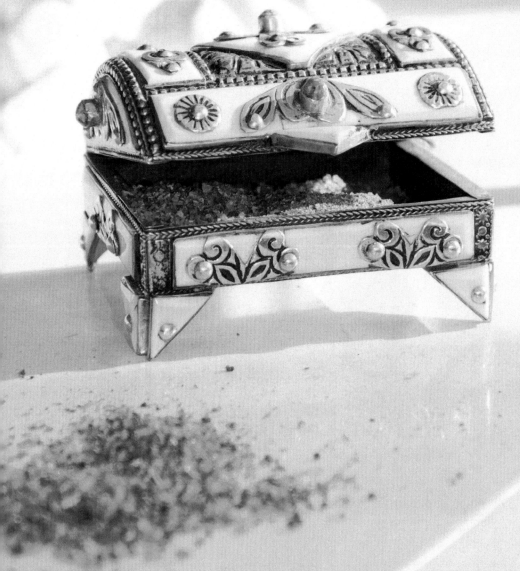

I won't panic about my bank balance when I go shopping, and I won't need to have long talks with my husband about how we will get through the next month. I won't be worried about how we can keep our family well. I will have energy for my day and for the people I love. I won't fear any new challenges that may come. I will drop everything and go see a friend who needs me if necessary. I won't regret that I can't help a charity I really want to help or support a cause I really want to be a part of. I won't still be wondering if I have what it takes to do something great in the world. I won't wonder if I really do matter and if the things I've been through have a purpose. I will think about people who need hope today for their wellness, and their finances and how I can spark the start of change for them. I will think about the awesome pleasure and responsibility I have to help other people see their purpose and fulfill it. I will decide to take a trip to see a faraway friends or family members. I may decide to rent a vacation house for some much needed R&R with my family. I will have the time to plan a service trip uninhibited by finances to help those I dream about helping.

Today I will learn new things and continue to grow as a person and a leader because of the tremendous opportunity that God has given us through essential oils. The combination of financial freedom and wellness open up more time and remove serious barriers to doing the things we feel most passionate about with that time.

None of that could be said about me just five years ago.

I have had some fabulous life experiences and some not so fabulous ones growing up. My early years started out in a small home in southeast Ohio. We lived a short stint in Florida, too, where I learned how much I loved sunshine. I certainly came from humble beginnings. We didn't have much. As a teen, through what can only be described as miraculous intervention, I had the opportunity to travel to many countries with a youth organization that exposed me to many extremes in impoverished places. My heart had become sensitive to the many issues around the world, and I knew that one day I wanted to make a very big difference. As I grew up and settled into adulthood, those dreams became like faint memories that were at times too painful to think of because of the improbability of any of them happening.

When it came to natural things, I used to be a skeptic. I used to think that since natural plants were not regulated by the powers that be that you could never really trust them. Instead, I basically turned into a human drug trial and I swallowed blindly for many years in spite of the side effects. I started paying better attention when I became pregnant with my first child. My struggles controlled me for about eight years before I finally realized I needed to do something different, and being responsible for another life was the catalyst for that change.

As an answer to my desperate prayers, I learned that what was going into my body had a lot to do with my struggles. I started to support my body's systems by changing my food to a more basic, natural, "common sense" way of eating. I decided that eating things as close to the way God made them as possible made good sense. I went for it, even growing my own food at one point. After changing what I was eating, purging crazy chemicals in our cleaning and bathing products, and using natural alternatives to support wellness, I had turned a huge corner. This in itself was a miracle. This encouraged me greatly because I started to believe that my body could heal itself and thrive again with support.

Essential oils arrived into the picture of my life and turned out to be the missing puzzle piece. Just one drop of essential oil during my first class and I was a believer that these were special and amazing. I couldn't believe it. In the end, it was a drop of essential oil that blew me away? I was curious and wanted to know everything about these particular oils since I had used so many before in my massage practice without the same impact.

I devoured information and read about the history of essential oils, which have been around for many thousands of years. I even read a chemistry book (a miracle since I really bombed chemistry in high school). As I learned, I was excitedly sharing what I knew with others. I was trying oils on my family and everyone I came across, seizing every opportunity to present a bottle of essential oil and rub it on someone! Sometimes that got to be a little scary for those who were still on the fence. But I persisted despite the rolled eyes and worried looks. I eventually learned to tone it down a notch!

I used to be afraid of speaking in front of others and unsure of whether I had anything to offer. After all, I was a broke and worn-out, busy stay-at-home mom who was often too dazed to remember what time I was supposed to be somewhere. I was just trying to stay alive and brush my teeth in the morning and shower. I had traded in giving therapeutic massages for wiping bottoms and playing peek-a-boo 24x7, which I loved but struggled with because of our financial circumstances. I was constantly torn about the feeling of needing to leave my babies and work outside the home, which is where I wanted to stay. My husband had a great international business, and yet it was not the right timing and it was shut down. He continued to work ungodly hours at his privately owned gym to make ends meet and pay our debts. We had the means to pay so there was no way he would allow us to file bankruptcy. The financial strain was unbearable. I was unsure how I would be able to continue purchasing the oils that made such a difference for me and for my family.

And so, when the business opportunity eventually came to light, it was a done deal. I knew I had to do it. When a product that is this amazing meets a business plan that is equally amazing, you can't lose. I was sharing anyway! Sharing with others was so easy because our intention was in helping them thrive in every aspect of life. I felt my purpose come alive in sharing a legitimate option for maintaining wellness. Because of this passion and sharing we were seeing rewards from the company and it was paying for our oils. That's when I realized that I should look at the compensation plan and become more intentional. I had the support of my husband and kids and there was no stopping. I felt it in my bones. I could see that the passion I had for one day, serving and helping many people, was going to get its moment. That moment came sooner than I thought it would as we found ourselves giving of our oils before we even had many to give. Once we recognized the need and saw that others wanted to be a part of giving with us, we pooled together and GiveOils.org was born. Essential oils have been generously donated to 22 countries in areas where there is desperate poverty and need from many wonderful people who also started following us on this journey. Those needs propelled me forward and getting to be a small part of fulfilling those needs gave me great joy and fulfillment.

Not only was my health thriving, I no longer felt helpless in contributing to our financial future. And I didn't wait until I knew everything or even owned every oil. I just started sharing. I was driven and fulfilled by the feeling of seeing others' lives change.

I gained confidence and belief that I could do this. My skepticism in network marketing was shattered when I came to realize the truth: In this business model, you succeed only by helping others succeed. I could stay at home with my children make a difference and earn an income all at the same time. I used the oils in everything from supporting our immune systems, cooking and cleaning, to making body products. Because it's a lifestyle, I didn't have to think of way to bring it up in a conversation. People could smell me a mile away, and that alone brought more interest. It's truly unbelievable how many people who have come into our lives and become like family to us as a result of simply sharing just one drop of essential oil. I'm so thankful for the friendship and camaraderie that comes when you build with relationships as your focus. This is truly what makes us wealthy, these relationships.

In our culture, we are basically bombarded by the constant stream of media and marketing that tells us what's "normal." It's normal in America to have many toxins on our lawns, in our homes, and in an air freshener plugged into the wall. But things are changing, and people want to be empowered and "in the know." It is a great feeling to be a part of something that is shifting what is normal and giving support for our amazing bodies a new priority. People want education. People are realizing they need to support the body and its systems to maintain wellness. People are willing to try affordable, natural, alternative ways. As people share their experience, the excitement and education is spreading across the globe. For me, I would have settled for just the physical well-being support. But the wonder of dōTERRA is that it sets up the opportunity for emotional, mental, and financial health for anyone who reaches for it.

The journey of the last five years has taught us many things, most of which was learned through our greatest failures and difficulties. Success is not birthed through one win after another; it's birthed through perseverance in one trial after another.

I've learned to enjoy the process of being shaped for the better by circumstances and issues that most people face while growing into their purpose and going after their dreams. You can choose which direction your circumstances will take you. I now stand on the stage with confidence and faith that I have something worth sharing—both my own story and these precious gifts of the earth. All along, dōTERRA was the avenue that brought our dreams back into the realm of possibility.

Essential oils are a special gift. They are a sign that we are truly loved from above. Being able to give of our time, talents, and oils has been one of the greatest blessings of being at this level. The thing about giving is that you become the recipient of far more than you gave. And it all begins with a single drop.

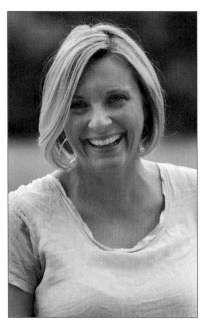

*Betsy Holmes is a wife, mom, licensed massage therapist, natural wellness educator, world traveler, philanthropist, and a Presidential Diamond Wellness Advocate with dōTERRA. She is a living testimony of not settling for less or accepting the status quo. Betsy's favorite part of being involved in network marketing is that she gets to use her life experiences, good or bad, to help people. Betsy's passion is to empower others to overcome challenges and fulfill their calling in life. Betsy and her husband Paul founded Give Oils.org as a nonprofit to use their influence and income to inspire change and healing for impoverished peoples around the globe. Betsy's faith, husband, and children are her inspiration for pushing herself to do the things for which she was born. She resides in Columbus, Ohio. **Learn more: www.gotoils.us, gotoils@gmail.com.***

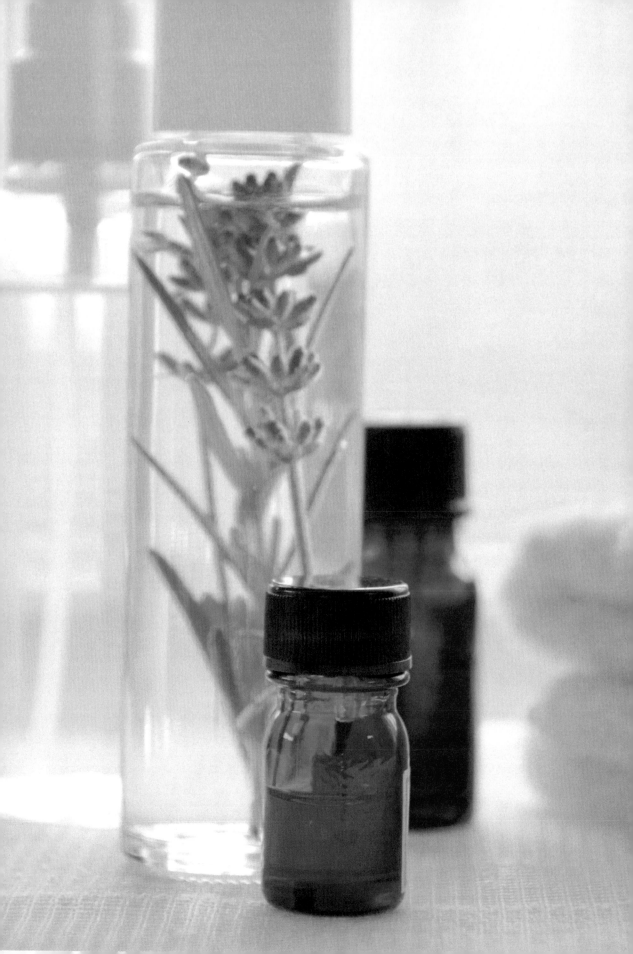

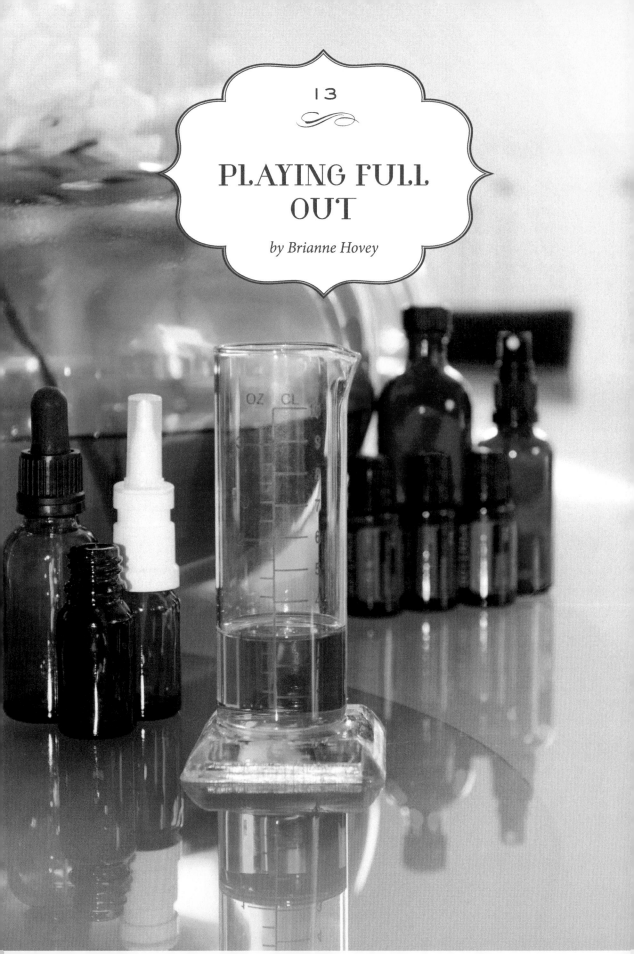

13

PLAYING FULL OUT

by Brianne Hovey

I grew up in a family where drinking green drinks and getting colonics was the norm. My dad owned a whole food company and my mom was into juicing and iridology. When I was ten, my mom was diagnosed with ovarian cancer. She passed away four years later. When my mom died, something shifted in me. I knew my purpose in life was to help others find solutions that aided wellness. I was adamant about making a difference and did not want others to experience the same pain and loss I had experienced at such a young age.

At age twenty, I dove into massage therapy and became an esthetician. I couldn't believe the healing doors that opened up! I loved getting my hands on others and seeing the transformation that happened in just one hour together. While doing body work, I learned that touch and personal connection are the most powerful healing tools we all have to offer.

That same year, I met Nate, and we married and had our first baby. But I was struggling, working in the corporate world for a company that required me to travel all the time when all I wanted to do was be at home with my son. During this crazy time, Nate lost his job, which added an insane amount of pressure on me to hold up the fort (that is, a $2,500 house payment). I was traveling for work and away from my son all the time. I became very depressed and could not see a way out.

I decided to take a leap of faith and quit my high-pressure, corporate job, with nothing in the pipeline waiting for me to catch my fall. I didn't have a plan B, I just knew I had to stop the insanity. We had been living in this paralyzing fear, extreme stress, barely making it paycheck to paycheck, drowning in medical bills, and having zero time together for way too long. We had had enough. As Jim Rohn would say, we had hit our wall of "disgust." We were finally asking more out of life and we were no longer going to settle for less.

I knew I wanted to remain in the health and wellness industry, I wanted to help others find natural solutions and make a positive impact in their lives. I wanted to wake up with purpose every single day. I found a job working at a wellness center near my home and was introduced to an incredible essential oil line. For the very first time I fell truly, madly, deeply in love with essential oils. I had never seen results like this with my clients before so I decided to take them home and use them with my family as well. I was so surprised what happened. Having the oils empowered us as parents. I felt in control as a mom, I could help my son in ways I never imagined and I knew we had found a solution to really help my family reach our health goals. These at-home essential oil experiences set a fire under us to learn all we could about oils. We now use them every single day. You might even call us junkies. My good friend once told me I have more oils than food in my house!

Funny how things work out in life. When we found essential oils we were thinking the oils were solely to help support us on our path to true, sustaining health. Instead, they would also become the vehicle in creating the life of our dreams. Ever had a single moment in your life that changed the fate of your entire future, a real honest to goodness paradigm shift? That moment was a phone call from my step sister, Allyse Sedivy. At the time I was working at the wellness center, barely keeping us afloat financially, and I answered a phone call that I will forever be grateful for. Within a one-hour conversation I knew everything was going to change. I mean *everything*.

Allyse asked me to become her business partner and create a business model around sharing essential oils with others. Although now I can clearly see this was a direct answer to my many prayers, in that moment I was scared. This was uncharted territory for me because I had never owned my own business before. I had never "managed" another human being. Leading a team of individuals flat out terrified me. But my belief in the oils and my dreams of being my own boss pushed me to jump all in. I wish I could write down all my stories. All the thousands of life-changing experiences I have had while on my journey sharing these powerful gifts of the earth with others. But instead I will share my top two lessons I have learned along the way.

Lesson number one: True joy comes when you are in the service of others. A spiritual leader of mine once said, "Forget yourself and get to work." I used to solely focus on me: my dreams, my problems, my stuff. Then I decided to shift my focus and put it on the people in my life. I really started to listen for every opportunity where I could help support someone with their health. I learned to be open and listen then *act* in the moments I felt inspired to serve. I made my business partners' dreams my dreams. I became fully invested in others' well-being and I forgot all about my problems and my excuses. In this process I found it is so much more exhilarating to watch my business partners' dreams come true than my own. The transformations that I have witnessed with the people closest to me, these soul-stirring moments, will be tattooed on my heart forever.

> *"You can have everything in life you want, if you will just help enough other people get what they want."*
>
> —Zig Ziglar

Lesson number two: Embrace the struggle. People are so quick to dream and so excited to succeed, but they want to jump right past the struggle. It ain't always easy to create the life of your dreams. When I started on this journey I seriously believed we would be financially free within eight weeks. No lie, and yes, it is extremely laughable at this point. Creating a dramatic shift in your life and getting a different result than what you are getting right now takes time! It takes hard work. It takes a ton of sacrifice and, most importantly, it takes discipline. I had to learn to master my mind. Those doubting thoughts can be sneaky, and they will find a way in and run your life if you let them. I had to focus on my talents and the greatness inside of me and stop focusing on all the negative lies. I now encourage others to start believing in themselves and *act* now on their dreams. It is in us. It is in every single one of us to live the life we were put on this earth to live. Play full out. Don't wait. Don't give up. You *will* get there.

This journey has been more fulfilling and life transforming than I could have ever dreamed. My amazing husband and I are literally living the life of our dreams *together,* and are leading the way for tens of thousands of others to do the same. We have teamed up with like-minded people who inspire us on so many levels and who are driven to make a difference. People who practice servant leadership and are passionate about giving back. We have a way to truly, physically connect with other human beings in sharing these oils. We need more of that in this world, and this is the vehicle to do it. My seven-year-old recently asked, "Mom, what do people do without essential oils?" My thoughts exactly, son.

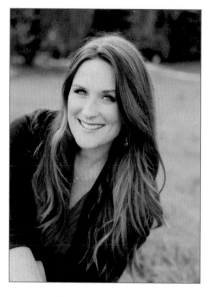

Brianne Hovey has over 15 years of experience in the health and wellness industry and holds the rank of Double Diamond in dōTERRA. She started her career in massage therapy and esthetics. As a National Educator she traveled to hundreds of spas teaching hands-on thera-pies and product knowledge to spa and wellness practitioners. In 2013 Brianne graduated from the Institute of Integrative Nutrition as a Holis-tic Health Coach. Brianne now travels around the world with her husband, Nate, holding nat-ural solution workshops and teaching individ-uals how to be self-empowered. Together, Nate and Brianne created The 14-Day Detox, *which includes the many benefits of essential oils. Bri-anne is the creator of the largest online Health Summit,* **naturalsolutionshealthsummit.com,** *and is asked to speak about natural health and personal development at large conferences around the world. Her passion lies in helping every person she works with discover their purpose and start living the life of their dreams.* **Learn more: www.essentialoilrevolution.com.**

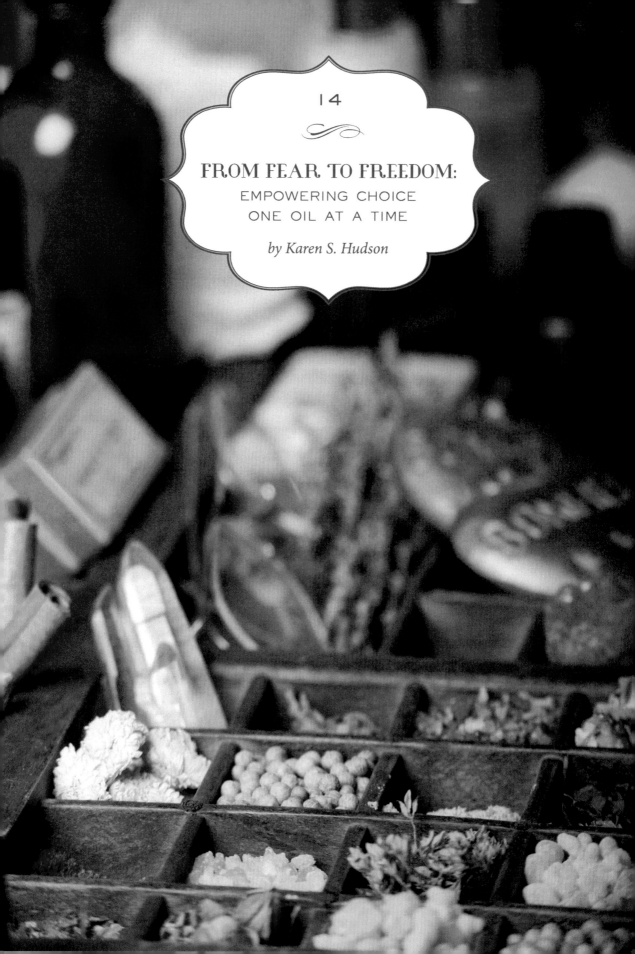

14

FROM FEAR TO FREEDOM:
EMPOWERING CHOICE
ONE OIL AT A TIME

by Karen S. Hudson

WE ALL HAVE PIVOTAL MOMENTS IN OUR LIFE—THOSE SECONDS THAT CHANGE OUR LIVES FOREVER. WE USUALLY FEEL LIKE THEY ARE JUST THAT MOMENT, BUT IN TRUTH THEY ARE THE SUMMATION OF A LOT OF SECONDS, MINUTES, AND USUALLY YEARS.

I was born into a house and family of chaos and confusion. My dad was an alcoholic and very angry man, and my mother was a very codependent woman who needed the appearance of her life to look better than the inside truth. Abuse, chaos, love, nurturing, fear, stuckness, and never talking about emotions or the elephant in the room—that was my home and family. All of it. I know my parents loved me unconditionally. And yet all of us kids were put through the wringer, and we were all affected by it in different ways. I became the person who acted out and said everything that came to my mind. I was the baby of the family and came in rocking and rolling—I definitely rocked the boat amongst the quiet chaos and abuse that was occurring.

I left home at sixteen and had my daughter when I was eighteen. The moment she came into the world I was changed forever. Given the role models I had, I was young and ignorant about how to keep my focus completely on her. However, even when she was young I could see she was different. Something was happening and I couldn't get a handle on it. By the age of four she was burning toys, throwing all the dishes in the house, and cutting things and she began to hit me. During these years I had begged borrowed and begged some more to send her to eight different treatment programs. She was kicked out of every daycare and class she was ever in. Teachers were scared of her, kids were scared of her, and I felt like I was chewing through concrete to save her, help her, and fix her.

My daughter's abuse toward me became stronger and more frequent. I was afraid of her. I slept with a knife under my pillow and in my purse every night and day since she was eleven. I was her mom. I gave birth to her. I wanted her. I loved her. I didn't know what to do, and through all of those years she ran away, was in a foster home, sent to treatment, hauled off the streets of the city, and became addicted to everything under the sun. I became the middle mom—the one that protected her from the world and the one that protected the world from her.

Fast forward to February 23, 2006. This is the day my first grandson Jack was born. My true healing began the minute I found out my daughter was pregnant. My mission shifted from her to him. I wasn't sure he would survive even the nine months in the womb. He did, thank goodness, and after a stint in the hospital, he came home.

For the first eighteen months, I tried to support my daughter in her parenting. And then, *my most* pivotal moment happened on December 8 at 4:23 a.m. That is the moment I knew I had to enact the safety plan and take myself and Jack to the safe house I had set up for more than a year. That moment—that decision—was the moment that by saving Jack, I saved myself.

I spent the next few years unwinding the chaos and helping Jack do it, as well. I had put myself on hold somewhere years and years ago as a child, then as a young woman, and then as a mother. My health was suffering, my heart was aching, and for the first time my house was quiet and there was room for more. I began a journey of connecting with myself. I had been so disconnected, desperately trying to save my daughter for thirty-three years that my whole being hadn't been taken care of, really, ever.

After five years of unwinding, I was ready to tackle my life in a real way, head on. And I found the Institute of Integrative Nutrition (IIN). I completed the studies, and along the way, I discovered tools and products and that would support my family and my clients.

You see, in all the years of working to save my daughter, I had gone back to college, gotten a dual degree in Psychology and Communication, worked on my master's in Human Systems Theory, obtained three prestigious certifications from the creators of Neuro Linguistic Programming, received certification in Family Constellations Systems, and was trained and certified in the methods of Dr. Phil McGraw. I also completed five years of coaching studies and mastery from Rhonda Britten at the Fearless Living Institute and earned three levels of coaching certifications. When I reflect back on all that I accomplished, I know it was all about my journey. Every class, every certification, every client, every moment was leading me closer and closer to a true connection with myself and the courage and ability to make that decision that one night at 4:23 a.m. in the dark of the early morning.

I was also earning a living through co-owning a women's natural health clinic, called A Woman's Time, with my sister. My journey with herbal supplements, tinctures, and essential oils began when I co-founded that clinic with her in 1995.

As I graduated from IIN and began taking on new clients, I was introduced to a new quality of essential oils. I had only used them aromatically and knew they could make you "feel good," yet really had no idea the true value of them. Being the researcher that I am, I decided to take on the task of exploring three different companies. After nine months of research, I made a decision. I knew which company and which person I wanted to align myself with. I enrolled. I knew I wanted to use oils in my practice with clients, and I knew I wanted to explore the possibilities of what oils could do to support the emotional and physical issues Jack and I had. What I didn't know was the impact the oils would have and how they would truly change our lives.

I feel like everything I have studied, lived through, and chosen led me to the point of this decision to change our lives and support others to create the life they yearn for, too. I desperately wanted to know if I could create an income doing something I love and am passionate about. How would I create this new cohesive way of living and being in business for myself?

I worked hard to know my own voice, to learn that I had the right to have it and have it be honored, yet I had to honor myself first. My entire unwinding was changing my whole life from the inside out. My journey with essential oils has been the gas that was finally put into the machine to make it fly. That machine is me.

I am creating a home filled with love, raising my grandson in peace, and breaking the chains that bound us both. From the day I opened my enrollment kit and began detoxing our lives from all toxic substances in my home, as well as detoxing our bodies and hearts, our lives have been forever changed. We are healing by doing the hard emotional work, and we are supported in that journey with essential oils and holistic products.

Being able to create a life for Jack and I means not only huge things for him but it helps me to create a new place for myself. My own feelings of worthlessness and helplessness have forever been rewritten. I now know I can create an income to support us comfortably—and, honestly, way beyond what I could have imagined. In two years I have surpassed the income I receive from my clinic. That is powerful! I now know and *believe* I can create what I need, and the possibilities for our future are endless. I have also been given the opportunity to realize new gifts within myself and how to use them. I love the team aspect of network marketing. I love mentoring, supporting, guiding, and leading others. I love that I can support others to reach for and obtain their dreams, their visions, and their desires. That is empowering to me.

Essential oils and the people I connect with every day have forever changed my life. And now I get the opportunity to mentor and support others to change their lives in the same way—fully, and from the inside out.

Anything and everything is possible.

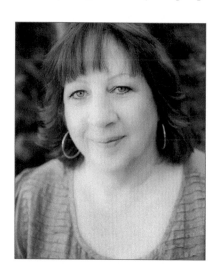

*Karen Hudson, CHHC, CFLC is a Board Certified Health and Life Coach, counselor, speaker, single mommapreneur, aka freedom fighter, fear slayer, and deeply compassionate champion/mentor. She is the founder and CEO of Change From the Inside Out, LCC, where she works with her clients to STOP THE WAR WITHIN˜ whether it's the battle with their fears, thoughts, beliefs, or bodies. From Karen's own personal journey through chaos, she now helps others create the life they crave and teaches how to live a life FULLY INSIDE OUT.˜ Karen's passion and love comes out fully with mentoring and building her team The Compassionate Oilers. The philosophy she teaches her private clients and her team is to meet people where they are. Karen asks the right questions, listens, supports, teaches, and guides them to manifest their dreams. **Learn more: www.karenshudson.com; Karen@ changefromtheinsideout.com.**

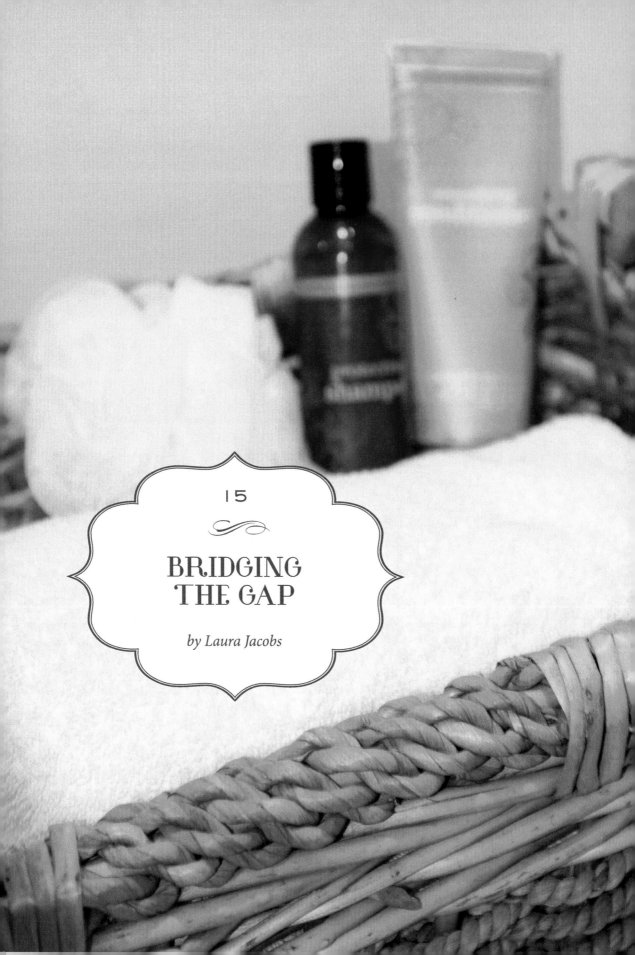

15

BRIDGING
THE GAP

by Laura Jacobs

While traveling in Jamaica, I loved what a tour guide told us. In her beautiful accent, she said, "Here we have no problems, only situations." Whether we believe we have a problem or we're caught up in a situation, no worries. It's life! We're just learning how to bridge the gap from here to there. The real challenge is being okay with the process—and being willing to learn from it. Each day, life serves up new lessons to chew on and digest. From these we can absorb greater truth and the knowledge and skills we need to make our dreams come true.

An easy life *is* a myth. Being *at ease* with life, however, is not. I've learned that when a situation arises, *any* situation, I have a choice about my response. Viewing life as a "classroom" and "situations" as teachers with lessons to offer has helped me be more at *ease*. Fighting against reality has only proven to be a rejection of precious opportunities to learn and grow. It takes authentic trust in the process called *life* to truly see things this way. Because embracing discomfort is the essence of being teachable, I've learned to invite myself to surrender. The result is I feel safe and more comfortable in my life, my body, my relationships, and my business ventures.

One of the main principles I've learned and use to guide my life and my dōTERRA business is that of *living the question*. This practice was inspired by the following words from Rainer Maria Rilke:

"Be patient toward all that is unresolved in your heart and try to love the questions themselves. Do not now seek the answers which cannot be given you because you would not be able to live them and the point is to live everything. Live the questions now."

—Rainer Maria Rilke, *Simple Abundance*

These words resonated deeply within me when I first read and contemplated them.

Over the years I've learned to love living the questions and to be patient as I make space and become ready to receive the answers. I've learned that whenever I feel there is a gap between where I am and where I want to be, that asking questions and believing the answers will come, is *my* part to do—not trying to dictate how the questions will be answered, or even whether or not the questions *will* be answered. As I've learned to detach myself from the need to control outcomes, I discovered that I can always trust the process, no matter what.

Surveying my past has been of tremendous value in order to discover the gaps in my belief, knowledge, and skill so I could build bridges to who I wanted to be. As I reflect on my childhood and youth now, I don't recall any noteworthy tragedies. I grew up in a nice, middle-class family and home with good parents. They were children of the Great Depression who chose to make a better life for their family. Hard work and service to others were core values I was taught in their household. They gave their children a tremendous amount of freedom and extraordinary trust, which was generally more common in the 1960s and '70s.

For me, however, trusting myself and life and the world around me was a work in progress well into my adulthood. When I was a little girl, I was inordinately shy in public. For those who know me now this is surprising! But for that little girl, whether being left at kindergarten or with a babysitter, the absence of my mother and being alone with strangers or lesser-known people was initially traumatic. In elementary school, I remained timid, sensitive to unkind acts from peers, and cautious about making friends.

Interestingly, when it came to the people in my inner circles, I felt very different. When I was with my siblings, cousins, and neighborhood friends, I was terrifically adventurous, leading endless hours of play at home or in parks, in our swimming pools, at the beach, or roaming miles of creek beds with these other kids both behind our home in California and in the rugged, rattlesnake-ridden mountains of Southern Utah we visited during numerous family vacations.

Life was good and relatively simple. It was hard work and dedicated play. *Do it yourself* was the theme and doing everything with excellence was a self-perpetuated expectation. Nowadays we call that *playing full out*. We were expected to do all the necessary jobs to maintain home and yard. Similarly, we were left to do-it-yourself play without much supervision or coaching and we indeed *played* full out as well. Ours was a family that simply got the work done, most often each working independently, and without pomp and circumstance.

An important part of the fabric of my childhood was how I thrived on creating with imagination. From building Lego dwellings and drawing *numerous* house plans on large sheets of newsprint paper (I did eventually graduate to graph paper), to creating elaborate six-story homes for my Barbie doll on a bookshelf (using all kinds of odds and ends for furniture), constructing large families with cutouts from the Sears catalog, and building forts under the dining room table, I loved creating imaginary worlds with my friends, cousins, and siblings. Any place from a sandbox to a mountainside would do.

As a family, we weren't terribly sports minded. But there was one thing we did do more and more often as I grew older, and that was dreaming with my mother. Our life was good. But who doesn't dream of more and bigger? My mother was always a willing participant and often led in any imagining discussion, planning everything from opening a bed and breakfast to remodeling our house or purchasing a vacation home or boat. Dreaming of a better life was a serious family sport and I was genuinely enrolled in the pursuit and potential success of every idea.

It wasn't until decades later that my husband and I together realized that nearly none of these plans ever came to fruition and that it didn't really matter to my mom. She seemed to be satisfied with the joy of simply imagining and dreaming up a grander life.

I do have to confess that I had always found myself longing for something more—for some of those dreams to actually come true, although they seemed well beyond my reach. Rather unconsciously I set out to take charge of making something happen. My entrepreneurial instincts kicked in at the ripe old age of twelve, when I became responsible for buying my own clothes. That's important to a seventh-grade girl! I was motivated by needing money. I wasn't afraid to work hard to get what I wanted. I hired out my services to the neighbors and local church members for house cleaning and babysitting. By age sixteen, I secured a "real" job—not surprisingly, at a clothing store in the mall.

I wasn't terribly self aware, but the businesswoman inside me had awoken. Having a hearty work ethic and the ability to make an income was gratifying and a success that spawned greater self-confidence. Important to my story however is that fact that I spent much of my high school and college years suffering from a type of inward social awkwardness; a sense of being alone and disconnected prevailed despite being surrounded by bright, charismatic, and popular friends. Outwardly and socially I successfully navigated my way without much difficulty. Inwardly, however, certain shyness still prevailed where I often was the observer more than the participant. I didn't perceive myself as a qualified leader so I acted more as a follower than an influencer. This sense of disconnection is a profound foreshadowing part of my story.

After my college years, and not yet married, I naturally focused on successful employment. Sales were my forte. I enjoyed the competition of being the top performer. From young adulthood and into my early married years, from working in retail clothing sales, to selling roofing, running a hugely successful vendor service business, selling life insurance, and being an event planner for a Senate campaign, no matter where I worked or what I did I loved the challenge of performing and being rewarded financially for my efforts. Developing this aspect of myself was critical to the success I would later experience in owning my own wellness business and building a successful dōTERRA team. Despite complaining like any child when given chores, my childhood had instilled in me a work ethic that had gone beyond habit. It had become a part of me. It became my character. All of these situations were indeed my classroom serving up numerous moments of preparation for my future. Who I would become was very dependent on what I did then.

Within months of getting married, I realized I was tired of working for someone else and jumped on an amazing opportunity for self-employment. I have rarely held a 9-to-5 job thereafter. Since then, I've started successful businesses over and over again, each time discovering more about what I was naturally good at and what I could generate with commitment and determination.

At twenty-eight, my sense of vitality and health began to diminish from years of neglecting myself and overworking motivated by ambition. In searching for solutions, an entirely new world then opened up: the world of natural health. At first, I sought experts who could teach me how to lead a healthier life. I read books, lots of books. I sought training. If I couldn't find or afford for someone to teach me, I taught myself concepts and modalities. In some cases, I bartered my time for the cost of tuition. I was enthralled, passionate, and driven to experience more, learn more, and share more. Natural health and wellness became a growing part of who I was and how I thought. Experiencing compromised health and the pursuit of solutions radically changed my life and that of my family forever.

My love of learning and willingness to share it continually landed me in moments where I was esteemed an expert in my field, spurring me on to eventually own a successful wellness center for more than eighteen years and accepting or creating numerous opportunities to speak and teach. I spent tens of thousands of hours serving tens of thousands of people and built a community of like-minded individuals who trusted me. This season of my life, serving as a health coach and educator, was wonderfully rewarding and terrifically satisfying. I loved creating problem-solving methods to better my services and, most of all, I loved helping people discover solutions.

Despite all this, as the years progressed, I often felt a gap between where I was and where I wanted to be. I knew there was more. I knew I was to move beyond providing one-on-one services and grow to lead a cause. It was during these years that my motto "A Healer in Every Home" was created and that I set the outrageous goal of affecting one million households. I rarely hesitated to accept opportunities to expand and grow my influence. They came fairly often but never materialized into what I envisioned they would. Just as in my childhood, I longed be part of a grander scheme that I knew in my gut would be part of my personal progression. The lack thereof sometimes frustrated me and I joked that I had been pregnant with myself for nearly ten years and could not deliver the "baby."

In retrospect I believe my longing for something more persisted because I had yet to truly experience who I am. Not who I am by my own construct but who I am by divine design. As Margaret Young once wrote: "You must first be who you really are then do what you need to do in order to have what you want." Although wonderfully more advanced, far more self aware, and spiritually much more alive, that internal disconnection of my youth still persisted.

Without knowing, I was living the question: What am I intended to be and do while alive on this planet? I had developed superb skills and knowledge over the years and was using them to serve others to a point of excellence, but I wasn't yet functioning in my true zone of genius.

I've been quite the reader over the years, and the book *Simple Abundance* by Sarah Ban Breathnach was an important part of my journey. She subtitled her book a "daybook of comfort and joy," and it was exactly that for me: a source of comfort and joy. I read it daily, as intended, and repeated the process for a number of years. It made a significant impact on my thinking.

I loved the opportunity Breathnach gave me each day to pair her thoughts with any other reading I was doing and I enthusiastically accepted her invitation for daily introspection. Her writing always seemed to magically dovetail and to be just what I needed in the moment. As I reflect back on why the experience of reading a daybook was so valuable, I realize that it was a form of mentoring for me. What I was longing for all those years was companionship, someone to walk by my side and speak to me on my journey. Not someone to parent me, or criticize me but rather someone to befriend and counsel me, to ask me thought-provoking questions and allow me to find the answers I was seeking at my own pace and in my own style. Through her book, Sarah Ban Breathnach was that person for me. She helped me learn to listen—not periodically but continuously. I was learning to listen to truth. Not to her truth, just to plain truth. She played the role of the gatherer, placing small essays in front of me, like a meal, to ponder and digest and glean meaning.

In the beginning of *Simple Abundance,* Breathnach reflects on how she discovered that her main source of unhappiness was the result of not living the real life for which she was created, what she calls the *authentic life.* That notion resonated powerfully with me. Not that I was unhappy. I wasn't. But what I heard her speak to was my never-ending gap: the gap between who I was and who I thought I had been created to be, a persistent internal disconnection.

Today I know that my authentic self was waiting patiently for me to recognize her. By learning to live my questions, I was getting closer to finding her. One of the most powerful realizations that happened for me as I practiced my daily introspections was discovering that I lived too much in my future. Or, rather, I was attracting my future too early or before I was prepared to nurture or sustain it. Therefore, opportunities would fail or never come to fruition. They were amazing ideas that were unsustainable. Premature discussions and pursuits of my future were the creator of the gap! That childhood family pattern of ever dreaming, never actualizing was hindering my progress. I needed to *participate* in my own dreams-come-true, not just to think or talk about them. I needed to learn how to attract differently, to attract results not just ideas.

Part of this awareness was the cold, hard reality and chastisement that I couldn't *afford* my dreams. Literally, the cash flow did not exist to support them. I had a profound moment of being divinely knocked upside the head with this knowledge, which made me more determined to reel myself in and demand that I stay present and live in the now. I began living the question of how I could increase my cash flow while remaining true to my core values.

Shortly afterward, in August 2008, one of my best holistic health students and referrers of clients, Natalie Goddard, came to me with the opportunity to join a new essential oil company called dōTERRA. I quickly rejected the idea, feeling that I'd had too many network marketing and aromatherapy disappointments over the years. I assumed myself to "be past" anything of the sort and on to better purposes.

The *only* reason I have a story to tell you now is that shortly after I rejected Natalie's invitation I distinctly felt an instruction to "get over myself" and my past and listen. My instincts told me that the message deserved my attention and that I had something to learn from the messenger.

The rest, you could say, is history. And the rest *is* more of my grand story of personal development.

One of the greatest things I was told early in my years in dōTERRA was: "Above all else, network marketing is one of the greatest courses in personal development." Although it was easy to agree with the concept, I know so much better now the wisdom in those words.

One of the most poignant moments in my dōTERRA life was to experience intense rejection when I learned that speaking of, or dreaming of, success was not enough. The lesson of the gap had come again! I was told bluntly that only those who live success can teach it. One of the owners of dōTERRA saw something in me early on that I did not see in myself. But, after a season of waiting on me to become the required rank for certain opportunities, he let me know that I was to be passed over unless I hit the mark.

I heard his message loud and clear, though I can't say that I figured out how to succeed overnight. I was slow to let go of old roles at my wellness business. I was slow to assume new ones. It was easier to acquiesce to my upline leaders. I was sure they had the leadership thing figured out better than I did so I rode on their coattails, staying the comfortable downline "child." I was slow to assume a leadership role.

My breakthrough moment came when a fellow dōTERRA member gave me the gift of honestly reflecting to me how I operated. That awareness was life altering. He helped me see how I was *still* creating my own gap. Only this time it was different. He acknowledged that I knew who I was and what I was doing in my life's purpose. But he challenged me by asking, did I know how to help other people find theirs? Being my authentic self wasn't enough to help other people bridge *their* gaps to their own authentic selves! Having been awakened to my situation, I quickly and assertively assumed the helm of leadership in my team.

With the discovery of what I needed to do, the success that had eluded me for years in dōTERRA was mine nearly overnight. When the student is ready, the teacher appears. My awareness was followed by intention and taking clear, precise actions. From the day we spoke, I accelerated through the ranks from Platinum to Diamond in three months, to Blue Diamond in just three more, and on to Presidential Diamond in twelve more months. Critical to this success was the fact that the leader of each new leg literally came to me and asked to build a dōTERRA team.

Certainly there were failures at every turn. Certainly there were setbacks. But really that isn't the story I want to tell. Why? Because I never let them stop me. That work hard, do-it-yourself, play full out, and "do so with excellence" character embedded deeply within me prevailed and trumped any discouraging situation. They really were only *situations,* not problems. They were feedback. They were lessons. Failure was my teacher. If something didn't work that meant a better way needed to be created.

I consistently recognized gaps in training and actively participated in creating solutions by collaborating with my direct upline, corporate owners, fellow leaders, friends, and members of my downline. Together we problem solved. Together we made things happen. Together we sacrificed.

I felt divinely warned not to allow my gaze to be distracted. I was continually reminded to *stay the course.* Never before in my life had I mastered how to nurture present moments while trusting that future dreams would indeed come true. And now, with dōTERRA's opportunity, they were coming true and far beyond what I ever thought possible.

Trust the process. Anyone who knows me well knows that I live by these words and as if my life depends on it, because it does. These words comfort me and invite me to be at *ease*, even when it's difficult. I live by them because they remind me there are never problems, only situations, only lessons.

As Rilke wrote, "Be patient toward all that is unresolved in your heart" and learn to love the lessons themselves. "The point is to live everything." Live the lessons now. The lessons are the course of personal awareness, development, and mastery.

And why would we develop ourselves? To bridge the gap to our authentic selves and to manifest the full measure of our creation! To share our gifts, skills, knowledge, and abundance as servant leaders who change lives and make a difference on the planet. Join us in this great cause.

Thank you, dōTERRA, for being a vehicle through which I could discover and manifest what I always knew was within me. Thank you, to my maker, for the gift of life itself, for divine guidance—for lovingly and patiently guiding me on my path so I could overcome my fear of the authentic greatest that was divinely planted within for the purpose of serving in the world.

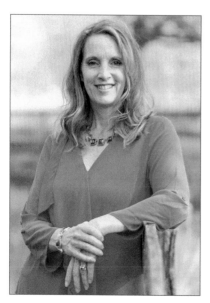

Laura Jacobs is a wife and mother of five and has served for decades as a wellness educator, international speaker, mentor, author, and a previous wellness center owner. She is the founder and leader of the global movement A Healer in Every Home, joining her purpose with dōTERRA wellness advocates whose collective passion is changing lives. Laura has taught thousands of health enthusiasts how to be the brilliant solutions providers in their own homes by empowering them to take charge of their diet, lifestyle, and individual and family health and wellness decisions. She loves family time and traveling the world with her husband and children, being an active member in her church and community, and living on purpose. **Learn more: laurajacobs.com; laura@laurajacobs.com.**

THOUGHTS ON
LEADERSHIP

by Laura Jacobs

Many of the leaders in dōTERRA attended a leadership event in March 2015 where the keynote speaker was therapist and author Connie Podesta. Among many entertaining and thought-provoking remarks, Podesta shared a profound concept that struck a chord in me. She talked about three kinds of people we could expect to interact with in our network marketing organizations: the top 30, the middle 40, and the bottom 30.

The top 30, she said, make things happen on their own, so they won't really want or need a lot of support from an upline leader or mentor. They can however be wonderful collaboration partners where their own talents and gifts are given place to shine and create results.

The middle 40, she taught us, is where we should focus our efforts. Why? Because these people are sincerely hungry for success but lack the skills or know-how to make it happen. They need support so they can gain the skills and mindset necessary for success.

The bottom 30, she said, operate from hurt and anger and use those to manipulate and guilt others into making success happen for them.

She counseled that most of us waste too much time trying to support the top 30 and the bottom 30. Instead, she said, we should focus most of our attentions on the middle 40.

After I left the leadership event, I shared this concept multiple times because I found value in its wisdom. As I pondered it further, it then dawned on me that we *all* have a bottom 30, middle 40, and top 30 within us that show up in how we run different areas of our lives. Each of us chooses where we operate from on any given day, in any given moment, and in the management our dōTERRA businesses. We can ask ourselves, "Am I functioning as my best, most resourceful self as a builder and leader?" "Am I hanging back and being less active than I could be in my own success?" "Am I waiting for someone else to hand me the results I desire or do 'it' for me?" Or, "Am I fully engaged in the process of creating my own success?"

Often we are hanging out in our middle 40 due to lack of skill, knowledge, or attitude. These are all parts of our second nature and what we establish as habit. Building a business and team in dōTERRA naturally provides a safe environment where one can experience a gradual or rapid growth in these areas. The more we do certain behaviors we move beyond habit and they can become a more natural part of our character, in essence becoming who we are and how we operate.

If you find yourself choosing to operate in areas of your life from your bottom 30, "using" and exaggerating the tragedies of your life to manipulate results, I share this: You can choose to experience life's moments and lessons tragically or triumphantly. Will those moments become an excuse for mediocrity or an unsatisfactory life? Or will you accept the lessons wholeheartedly and embrace them as precious moments to be taught so you can learn and grow and become? Your past holds your future captive. Let it go. Rewrite it. Your top 30 awaits you!

If you are someone operating from your middle 40, identify your gap, then build a bridge by getting trained and mentored. Your initial goal is to become consciously aware of what you don't know. Identify the skills you lack and pursue the appropriate education. Form new habits by training your mindset and skillset and gaining knowledge about your business and products. Make personal development part of your daily practice. Observe the skills and attributes of those who operate in their top 30 and aspire to acquire them. Learn them. Practice them. Very few people are born operating in their top 30. Nearly all acquire it. The position of being in the top 30 percent and most successful in any endeavor is the result of practice and doing specific things consistently until those things become part of who you are and what you do.

If you are truly, consistently operating from your top 30 percent capabilities, kudos! You are likely experiencing your authentic life. The pages of this book are filled with examples of inspiring women who have discovered the secrets of success and authentic living.

Interestingly, one of the greatest challenges for the successful top 30 is to identify their unique formula for success. You may tend to operate from what is called *unconscious competence,* meaning that you don't fully know why you are successful. It's become such a natural part of how you function. If this is the case, you'll be even more wildly successful if you can identify certain core principles and teach others how to follow a proven system of duplication and allow for *their* unique gifts and talents to shine through.

It's one thing to be a guru; it's another thing to support others in the process of discovering and becoming their own success stories. With dōTERRA, true servant leadership drives success: No one succeeds alone. When we can inspire and empower others to find the path to their successes, that's when we've really cracked the code of creating the world, the business, and the lifestyle we want to live in. The transcendent path of serving others is the true path to happiness and self-actualization.

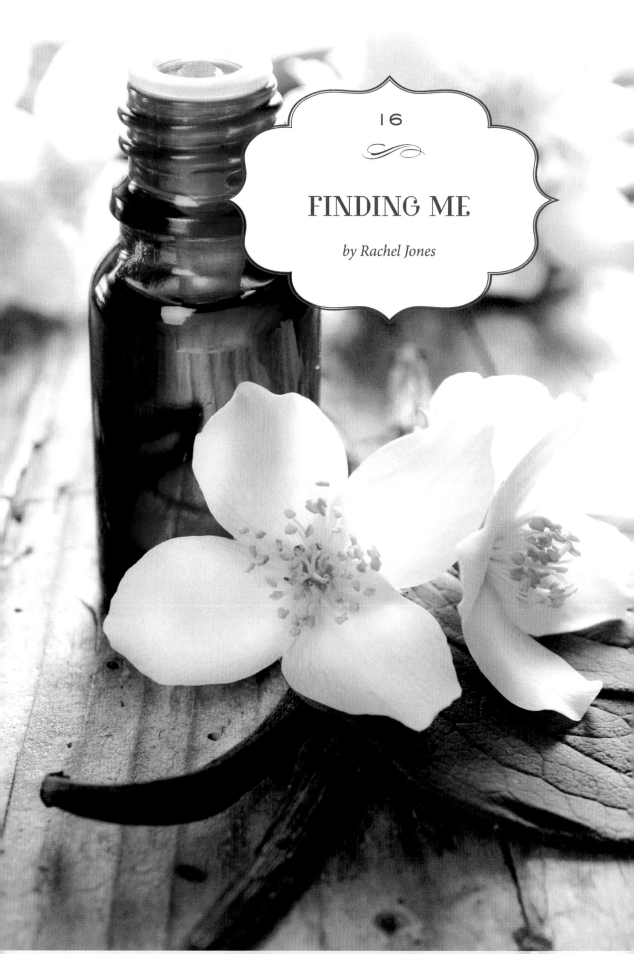

16

FINDING ME

by Rachel Jones

What was my secret to never failing, and being so easily successful?, I was asked. In that moment, I laughed out loud and wondered how I had gotten away with being so perfect in other people's eyes. That is not even close to how it has looked on my side of the mirror.

In January 2014, I was in Tulum, Mexico for dōTERRA's incentive trip with my husband, who was still working outside of the oils business at the time. I was about to launch my first retreat along with so many other heavy responsibilities. But, for months, I had been having a growing feeling of being lost. I kept thinking something needed to change, and I was desperately trying to figure out what I needed to fix in my life or change in my business. I did energy work, worked with coaches, worked out, ate clean, and set aside time with my kids… Why was I feeling so lost? Worse, this feeling kept growing, no matter what I did.

On the trip, I reached out to a dear friend and leader in my company. I told her, "I need to change how I lead my team because I think their growth is stuck."

She directed me to the book *The 21 Irrefutable Laws of Leadership* by John C. Maxwell and Steven R. Covey. The law that came up for me was Nine: the law of magnetism—who you are is who you attract. The book stated, "Believe it or not, who you attract is not determined by what you want. It's determined by who you are."

Well, that just made me mad. I wanted my leaders to look a certain way and do what I wanted them to do because that was how they would be successful. And it just wasn't working. What was wrong with them?!

As I calmed down and looked at my accountability and why I was so mad, I realized the problem was with me. If who I was wasn't someone I liked, who would I attract? Major introspection followed. My internal paradigm started shifting. I kept searching for answers about what to do next. How could I change things so they would just start working? While I was asking for the bigger perspective, I really just wanted to solve this problem with my team. It was all about how I could go Blue Diamond right now.

The last speaker that night sought me out to talk privately and asked how he could help.

I cut right to the chase. "How do I rank advance to Blue Diamond? What do I need to do?"

His answer was just as direct: "It isn't what you need to do, it is what you need to stop doing." He said, "Do less and connect with who you are more. Meditate and build a relationship with who you are instead of jumping to the next thing just trying to be successful. This training, that training—just stop! Work on you and you will hear what you need to do next."

I was thinking, "But what if it tells you to let go of your grip? Will all hell break loose, or do you just trust?" Still in resistance, I asked that question, never really wanting to just trust. Knowing that I was still missing the point, he tried again.

"Meditation will bring you to a new place you haven't visited inside," he said. "That will bring out the true you. Ideas will spring. The spiritual side of you will rise, which is actually the more powerful and knowledgeable side."

With his words, my body relaxed and my mind was able to let go enough to open me up to the beauty around me and to simply be present with the waves on the beach.

Now, honestly, my head hadn't let go of Blue Diamond. But my heart heard and felt lighter and peaceful.

I discovered that night that I had created this person who had been living in her ego. I was focused hardcore on the things I thought I could control. If I was Blue Diamond it would mean I was good enough. On top. Blue Diamond was who I wanted to look like.

I stood alone on the dark beach looking out at the sea and up to the stars, and I felt as if God was right there talking to me. I had been in so much turmoil and desperation about what I was going to do next, and my friend had spoken the truth that was already inside me that I wasn't hearing. At that moment, I felt the love of God so warm and loving. My heart was heard.

My husband, Brian, had come to Tulum on his own personal journey as well. I had wanted Brian to eventually come home and build this business with me, but up until Tulum he couldn't see how this could happen or even why he would want it to. That week, surrounded by supporting successful leaders, turquoise water, and the quietness far removed from the intense stress of his job, he saw why. So when I returned to our room that night and woke him up, telling him everything, he immediately felt the shift in my heart and understood.

I had come to Tulum flailing like a drowning woman. I left Tulum with new clarity, a book on meditation as the way to begin knowing myself, and a deep sense of peace and purpose. I was connected inside again.

But as I have come to realize, understanding doesn't change everything.

As the weeks passed, I found myself once again growing agitated and anxious, looking at my business and feeling frustrated. I still wanted Blue Diamond, and I was struggling to learn how to want to achieve a goal without it determining who I was to myself. My winning had always been part of who I am. I had never been in this place before, and I didn't like it.

It was looking like my dream wasn't going to work out, so I had to focus on other things and let Blue Diamond lie to the side. This killed me. I was constantly trying to stop myself from repeating the old pattern, which I ended up repeating anyway. My emotions spiraled downward into dejection, and I lost hope. At that point, I believed that my only two options were to force things by going all out like I had been doing, or give it up altogether.

We had a big victory during this time when Brian decided to leave his job of nearly thirty years leading a family business and work with me. I thought all my struggles would disappear and Blue Diamond would be in the bag. As you can guess, that isn't how it works. Again, I was trying to force.

I tried practicing meditation and was able to do it more regularly at first, but gradually I chose to do other more "immediate" things, and so my practice fell off. When I would try to go back to it, I would find myself agitated and unable to sit still. I couldn't focus to save my life.

Then at the beginning of July 2014, I was on a morning walk with a friend who is Blue Diamond. At her suggestion, we sat down to look at my organization and she showed me with the numbers how I could go Blue. Interestingly, through the spring I had let go of internally pushing my leaders so I could instead practice just listening and supporting. Without knowing beforehand, the result of this was unexpected changes and activity at just the time I decided to work for Blue. I had hope again.

With only July and August to qualify before Convention, I stopped forcing and started listening; I was going Blue Diamond.

But I couldn't do it without my team. I was nervous as I shared my dream with them and asked if they wanted to go for it too. This time I wanted to hear them, and as I listened to them and what they wanted, they said, Yes! Momentum was building. I was so excited—things were moving forward! I put incentives in place and worked with my downline to hold classes—I did everything I could think of.

But about the middle of the month as I looked at the numbers, my heart sank. I was so far away. Too far. And as it does when we open the door, discouragement set in. I saw my coach and laid out why it wasn't going to work. At first, she tried to get me to step back and connect with my vision. That had worked before, but this time I couldn't see it. I wouldn't see it. My push for Blue wasn't enough to make it happen.

Then out of nowhere, she said quietly, "Okay. Then quit! Walk away. I will love you just the same tomorrow. Everyone will still love you. We will still know what an incredible woman you are, and no one will blame you at all. You can go for it again another time, Rachel. You are free to walk away."

The silence hung between us, as my choice sat squarely in my lap. She reiterated what she'd said, giving me complete permission to step out. At that point, something inside me rose up against all that logic that told me it was a losing battle, that I should just walk away and try again another time when conditions were more favorable. Right then, this part in me decided I was all in, no matter what the outcome. I would not quit today.

I was on fire again, and as I worked with my team for their success, I saw them come together to support my dream too. The results were astounding, and as the month came toward its end, I saw miracles happen in legs below mine that had never happened in all the three years of my pushing and trying to create Blue.

With just days to the end of the month, I felt like I was on a tightrope keeping my head high and focused. I had been strictly controlling my negative thoughts from spiraling down so I wouldn't fall again. With seventy-two hours left, I looked at my numbers. They simply weren't there. I was sick inside. That afternoon, my hope was fast bleeding out. I prayed. Only this time, my prayer wasn't for the help to make my goal happen as it had so often been. This time, I came to my knees letting go. All I asked was for clear guidance whether I was to let go and stop or keep going. As much as I wanted this goal, I let go entirely in my heart to receive and accept exactly what was in front of me whatever it was.

I felt peace. And as I got up, some fresh laundry fell off the bed. Stuck to one article of clothing was the Blue Diamond pin that one of my sponsors had given me a couple months prior to show me how much she believed in me. I couldn't imagine how it had come to be there, but in that moment, I felt my body become so very light again as it had in Tulum. The very clear divine permission spread through me to let go, trust completely, and take it all the way. I knew that I would go to the end, no matter what the outcome. In my deepest desire, I had let go and listened. I was trusting.

Too many unbelievable events and miracles happened in those seventy-two hours to be able to recount them all here. But I can tell you that it came down to the final hours before midnight with crucial spots still uncertain and no way to check in with those people. I wasn't there by myself. Working together with Brian and with my leaders both in person and over the phone, we opened the door for miracles to happen. I did every single thing I knew to do. I let go, minute by minute, and pushed to the end.

It wasn't until 2 a.m. that I was able to see the final numbers. My leaders were Gold. I was Blue Diamond. We had done it.

As I listened to my friend who thought I somehow so perfectly met all my goals, and right on schedule, I told her I understood where she was. I had been trying to reach Blue Diamond for three years. I had felt there must be something wrong with me for not reaching my goal. I had made choices that didn't always look like they benefitted my children. I had pushed until I couldn't push any more. I had stayed up late, working hours that didn't seem to end and then starting again the next morning. Every Convention, I had felt inadequate that I wasn't farther ahead. So many people were passing me up because they must be smarter, more dedicated, better leaders…

But none of that was true. We learn who we really are by the challenges, both those we choose and those that happen to us. And my true goal, it turns out, was never Blue Diamond.

In the months that followed my walking the lavender carpet at Convention that year, I had a deeper inner peace. I had stopped trying to force, and I had really begun to learn how to listen. As I listened, I could actually finally hear me. All those feelings of not being smart enough, or a lousy leader, all the mental beating I had constantly given myself since I was young whenever I didn't win or didn't measure up by outside standards, it was being replaced by calm and peace more and more frequently. I was stopping the attacks on myself.

There were still the same struggles. There always are. We think we will reach "the goal" and everything will be different than it was. And I'm here to tell you, reaching a nearly impossible goal is incredible! It really is! But, for me, those goals aren't the real ones. And that is why all my attempts at "pushing" my goal to happen had been me fighting with myself. The deepest part of me had been patiently teaching myself to learn to let go and trust, quit trying to force: Listen. And in those quiet moments, I heard my truth. I am so incredibly loved. I am valuable beyond anything I had ever imagined in all the great successes of my life. I had found me.

So I will say, trust the process you are taking yourself on, especially when you can't see your way. That's when we really learn to listen. Something inside you that is not your head already knows the way. Know that when we begin to listen, the quest opens up wide as I recently discovered during a dōTERRA service trip to Guatemala with my whole family. I discovered yet an even deeper purpose for myself on the planet. This new horizon would not have been visible to me without the foundations I had painfully spent the past three years building. So know that the "outcome" is always only the next step. Don't stop, because it's your life you're actually living, not trying to "get to." And realize, there are so very many people we can and will help on our way.

We are happiest when we are in pursuit of our true dreams.
Trust me—everything is possible!

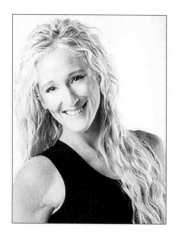

*Rachel Jones is a successful dōTERRA Leader and Health and Wellness Expert. Over the past two decades, Rachel has pioneered cutting-edge health practices in her community. Rachel and her husband, Brian, work their dōTERRA business together, are avid humanitarians, and travel with their children. You've seen her as the woman doing handstands—everywhere. Rachel is a Licensed Massage Therapist, Certified Yoga Instructor, athlete, and Natural Health and Nutrition Educator. Her life's work is to teach the integration of healthy life practices, mindset, and tools—including dōTERRA essential oils—to lift health to the highest levels yet. **Learn more: www.mydoterra.com/joy.***

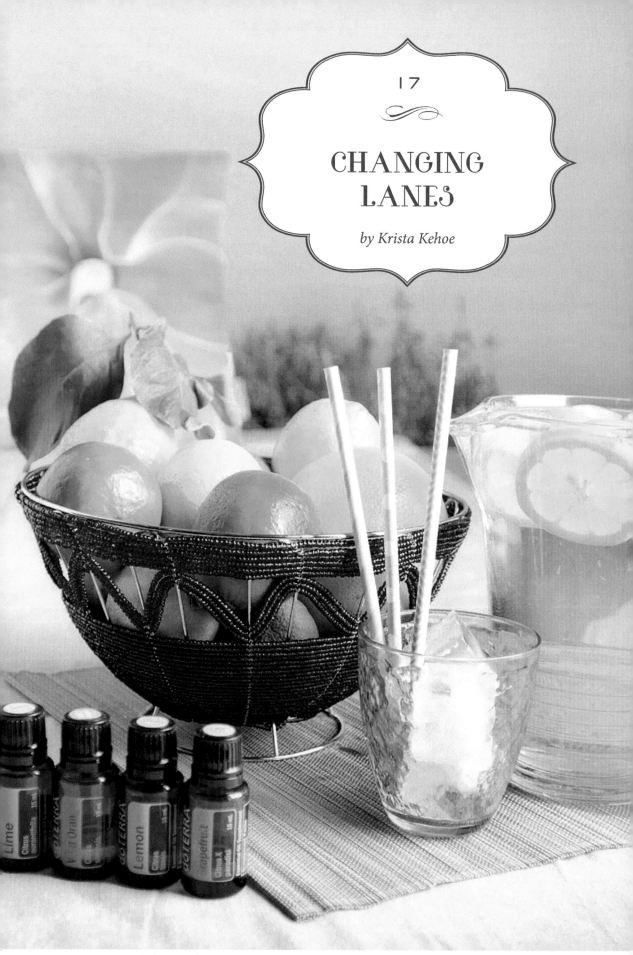

17

CHANGING LANES

by Krista Kehoe

With an affinity for health and wellness, I reveled in being "outside" and "all natural." I grew up with my horses in my backyard, and as a kid nothing was better than the time I spent breathing in the sweet smell of their energy. My dream was to have lots of horses and dogs and live a life that connected me to other living beings—including the four-legged variety!

I majored in biology in college and got my master's in Education. I made practical choices. I was taught that an education is the most important thing in the world; nobody can take it from you and from there you have more choices. But when I looked up from my work and my son was getting on the school bus without me as I headed out to teach before the sun came up, I realized that the choices I had given myself were no longer coming from a place of authenticity and happiness. I was tired and stressed and I didn't feel my lifestyle was sustainable for the long term. I needed a new strategy that acknowledged my role as a mom, my expertise in science and teaching, and my thriving interest in my horses, dogs, and fitness. This was my second or third wake-up call from the universe, and I knew it was time to listen.

Ten years ago I had my first major disappointment with our healthcare system. Nobody could figure out what was wrong with me until they realized my healthy intestinal flora had been wiped out by an antibiotic I had taken. I was young, miserable, and scared! So I began to investigate a holistic lifestyle. I tried acupuncture, Chinese herbs, organic foods, supplemental probiotics, essential oils, stress management and, as always, I worked diligently on my fitness goals. I learned so much about my body and how it can support itself when given the opportunity to be in balance. I learned to notice subtle signs of imbalance before they became full blown, and I gained confidence in my ability to be well and stay well. I was empowered to direct my health in ways that standard doctors weren't accessing.

The most powerful practice for me became nutrition, and the most valuable complement to my health and wellness was essential oils. But here I was a decade later and I wasn't happy with my current lifestyle and profession. I was living a very "secure" and tidy life as a teacher with a set schedule—doing things that theoretically made sense. But at my core, I was unsatisfied. I was so hungry to do something that made me light up and thrive. I had fought the urge to change careers for about eight years and had looked into several very viable options, but the Goldilocks in me found every excuse to stay where I was. The other possibilities were "too time-consuming" or required "another degree" or "wouldn't give me more time with family" or "would require a bigger commute." So I stayed. And I built resentment about what I "had" to do. I was living by the rules, but they weren't my own.

When I became a mom, I was lucky enough to stay home for my child's first year. I weighed the options and went back to work on the premise that everyone I knew really did go back! Only four months into daycare, my baby boy had pneumonia—twice. Not to mention the fact that he had been sick every other week with a fever since he had started daycare! That was it. My husband Kevin and I declared there would be no more daycare. So we hired a nanny and, after a time, even that didn't feel right. My gut said that this wasn't okay. Our son was exhibiting behaviors that came out of nowhere and I felt that I was away from him far too much. So Kevin and I decided I would take a leave of absence and I stayed home for two more years. Even though these two years were the most satisfying moments of my life, I was committed to go back, yet again, to work. After all, I was teaching in one of the top districts in the nation. My mindset dictated that I couldn't waste what I'd worked so hard for, and at my core I'd always felt that helping people reach their full potential was work worth doing. It felt like the right thing to do

I geared up to return to work and transfer my child to a new school with before and after care. But then, three weeks before I was to start, Kevin lost his job. In a strange way, I felt... relief. I knew our son would be able to continue at the school we thought we'd have to leave and that Kevin would be able to experience fatherhood in a way that so many dads don't have. So many wishes were answered. Over time, though, as I saw education continue to change, I realized I had lost my passion for changing a system that was outdated. I felt I was failing to meet the needs of all of my students in the process. And while I was at work, I felt like I was failing as a mother.

It was time to do some serious soul searching. I went to therapy where I talked about my passions, my lost purpose, my desire to be a mom—and my wishes to be secure at the same time. It was painful as I peeled back layer upon layer of fear. I added hypnosis to my regiment and then Reiki.

One day, I just stopped over-analyzing and I let myself feel what I had been afraid to admit. I had tried so hard to accept my current situation but it was time to make a change and there was finally a space in my life for it. But, even though I realized that the very thing making me feel secure—my job as a teacher—was squelching my light and my aliveness, I still didn't make a move. Looking back, I can hardly believe my tenacity!

I practiced yoga, read voraciously, and checked yoga blogs online to see what little pieces of enlightenment I could glean in my free moments. Out of the blue, I came across dōTERRA and researched it. It seemed too good to be true, and I thought it had to be a scam. But as I kept looking at the website and cross-checking references, I began to feel something familiar—I had felt it before when really good things happened in my life—when opportunities had presented themselves and I'd said yes and jumped in. Now I know that the term for this is "synchronicity." I talked to Kevin about the possibility of doing it as a business. I assumed he would be unsupportive, as I felt on the edge of crazy by that time! But he didn't bat an eye. He just went with it. I was scared to take the leap, because I knew I was making a big change in my life and it would affect all of us. But I walked right up to my fear and right through it and started my business.

In the science fiction film "Gattaca," there's a point where the main character turns to his brother and says, "You want to know how I did it? I didn't save anything for the swim back." He's referring to the idea that he jumped into something with all of his heart and didn't give himself an out. I started with the biggest business kit dōTERRA offered, and I didn't look back. There was no option for failure. Forty-seven days later, I hit the rank of Premier. After six months I was Platinum and a year later I hit the beautiful rank of Diamond. I took every second of mentoring that I could get from my upline sponsor.

I also enrolled at the Institute of Integrative Nutrition to become a certified health coach. This was something that had been suggested to me three years earlier and I hadn't followed up on it. It was another lead—another whisper—I had ignored.

My advice to you is to listen to that voice that continues to gently whisper to you. When you hear the same message from the universe two or three times or in different ways, open your eyes and check to see what you're missing.

I wish I would have started this journey earlier. It would have given me the flexibility to be home with my son from day one without sacrificing my role as a mother or my role as a professional. But, at the end of the day, I believe that the experiences I had as a result of working outside the home give me a unique perspective and drive for success that I wouldn't have had otherwise.

My flame has been fanned, my passion reignited. Ironically, my students had always known this was my passion. When I taught the units on basic biochemistry, they could always tell I was excited to share information about nutrition and wellness with them. They would ask me to talk about it for a full day! My students were one anchor—my "why"—and the reason I stayed in education. The other piece of my "why" was the salary and benefits it was providing to my family. However, by trusting my inner compass, I found that there was another way—a sustainable way—to use my expertise, be fulfilled, and live my purpose. Essential oils have given me this gift.

My essential oil business continues to grow, and I am inspired and mentored by other women who, like me, walked through their fears to live by their own rules in a world where it's easy to lose that choice. Although the process of awakening to my greater purpose included painful parts, and I sometimes felt that I was driving down a highway with my turn signal on, taking the leap is worth it.

Teaching continues to be what my life is about—my "why"—but now I teach on my terms with my rules. I work with intelligent, motivated women who also want to build their own businesses with essential oils. I've found a way to use my expertise and live my purpose. I now partner with people from all walks of life who are educated, vibrant, and open to new possibilities in their lives. As I interact with moms, career-changing adults, veterinarians, and animal professionals, I've found a way to apply my expertise in science and teaching with truly helping people access their best "self." I give back to the teaching profession—my roots—through a free program I offer to help educators reduce stress and lead more balanced and holistically healthy lives, *The Wise Balance Teacher Lounge*.

Yes, I even get to work with animals—my life-long dream. While changing lanes, I've found my bigger purpose and am able to explore something close to my heart. I now have the ability to honor all living beings with the oils, and I have access to an open road of every possibility that I manifest. I am finally in the driver's seat.

You have the power to be where you are and blossom or to bloom in a new place. It's up to you. If you listen to your inner compass, your higher voice and deepest desires, you will find your way, too.

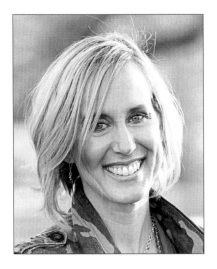

Krista Kehoe connects with and mentors intelligent women who get the concept that this life offers a finite amount of time and energy and finding what's essential is the secret to a life of holistic wellness filled with abundance, love, and happiness. She lives and loves with her husband, son, and pets in Iowa, where her business Wise Balance Lifestyle is exploding with growth and potential. When she's not mentoring her team or working on a bigger vision for herself, you can find her riding her horse or playing with her dogs, cat, and essential oils. If you are interested in a more vibrant version of yourself, or just want to check in and say hello, she's always on the lookout for new team members who bring their own set of strengths to the realm of essential oils and self-actualization. **Learn more: www. wisebalancelifestyle.com; krista@wisebalancelifestyle.com.**

"And the day came when the risk to remain tight in a bud was more painful than the risk it took to blossom."

–Anaïs Nin

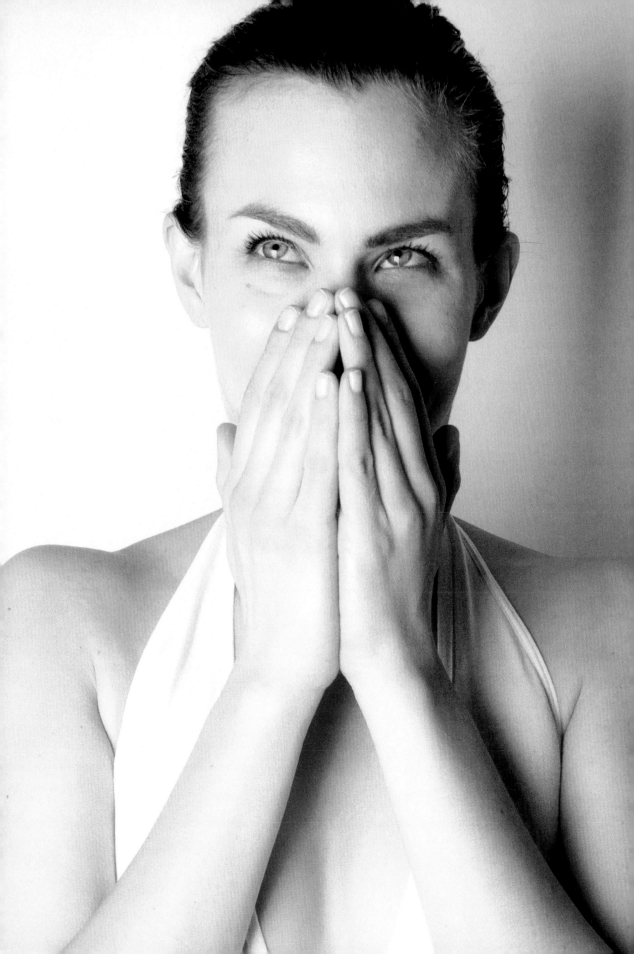

THOUGHTS ON
LEADERSHIP

by Krista Kehoe

I'm often asked what I did to achieve Premier rank within 47 days of my start date, Silver a month later, and Gold two months later... all while being "too busy" to work my essential oils business. I want people to know that it's really a matter of prioritizing. At the time of my oils "launch," I was waking up at 4:45 a.m., feeding my pets, working out until 6 a.m., leaving my house by 6:30 a.m. and working a full-time teaching position until 3:15 p.m. I didn't get home until after 4 p.m. at which time I was a mom and a wife. There was no "extra" time, but I forced myself to find the energy and I worked sometimes until 11 p.m. or midnight to get a handle on my business tasks.

How do you prioritize?

First, do the work of finding your "WHY." Start the process of branding yourself from day one. Of course, this process evolves over time, but the point is, get centered and clear about what you are doing.

Second, reach out to people in person or on the phone. Don't hide behind your computer and a bunch of evites. It's too easy to be ignored. Let people see your excitement and authenticity. Do not "sell." Share your experiences and expertise. Solve people's problems through the oils and products and opportunity.

Third, incorporate the oils into your life visibly. I used the products (and still do) religiously. It's not hard to do because I love them! At the gym, I pull out my Breathe™. At the barn, I use Peppermint. At my work I rely on Serenity and Balance, and I drink Slim & Sassy. People know I'm the girl with the oils.

Fourth, project confidence. When you're clear on what you're doing and the idea that something is worth it, it shows. I never for one second thought the products weren't worth it. I never said to someone, "Well, this is kind of expensive..." It's not for you to decide. Health is important. How can you put a price tag on someone else's health? I learned to put the offer out there and teach. And then I learned to be quiet. Let people think and make decisions for themselves. Show them the best value, and let them make an educated decision based on where they are at.

Fifth... do not let perfection stop you. When I first started, my upline asked when I would do my first workshop. "Workshop?" I thought, "I haven't even seen a class about oils being taught!" I thought she was crazy. Plus I had "no time." She reminded me that we are all busy and that the class was an hour of my time. I decided to be coachable, scheduled a workshop, and had ten people enroll. That was two weeks after I started with my company. You know what? She was right. I'm so glad I jumped right in or fear would have set in. Sometimes it's better to just get in and get your feet wet.

Finally, don't stop. You're going to hit roadblocks. So what? Everyone gets stuck from time to time. Don't stay there! Get back to your "WHY." At least these are the roadblocks you have chosen. That's why we have 4-wheel drive, right? Be creative. Get resourceful. Use your upline. This business is accessible to everyone. It's already proven itself. Use what is available to you.

People who succeed at this business go to training events, get on calls with their upline, follow suggestions, and duplicate the business. Take the coaching you are being offered! If you are coachable, your upline can help you. Be open. The truth is, if you succeed, so do they... so really, they have your back! What an amazing opportunity we all have to create our own reality and a stream of income from a focus on health and wellness. I can't tell you how grateful I am.

18

SAVING GRACE

by Rommy Kirby

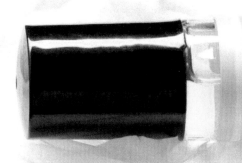

Each day was another day that I watched my children grow, explore, and live their lives without me. I was no longer able to sit on committees or chair foundations. I couldn't even go the movies with my children. Eventually, I gave up singing in the choir, teaching youth Sunday school, and rocking babies in church. The only joy I could find was in seeing my children grow and thrive. But even this, was without me. I was an observer.

To see me in public, you would never have guessed that I was so ill. I put on an Oscar-worthy show of vibrant health and happiness for just a few hours only to go home, lock the door, collapse onto my bed, and seek silence as tears fell down my face with shame, guilt, and pain. I searched from doctor to doctor for answers. The only answer they could give was, "We don't know what's causing this but you can take this pill"—and I might need to take them for the rest of my life.

In 2005, just as I was reaching the end of my rope, I found a physician who gave me hope and tools to change my health. My doctor understood holistic health and that one system relied on the other. He listened when I said, "I feel like I'm toxic. That there is something in my body that shouldn't be there." Together, we worked supporting and nourishing my body so that my body could release toxins the way it should. I changed my lifestyle from one of fake and fast convenience-style food products to one of whole foods, sustainable life supporting habits and products. In his office, I was introduced to essential oils.

You see, I really was toxic, or perhaps poisoned is a better word. I was the person with bleach stains on her cuffs and at her waist. I reveled in the fresh, clean smell of bleach. My hands and nails were always cracked, sometimes bleeding from harsh chemical cleaners. I hated germs and did everything I could to never ever come in contact with them. I had breathed in so many cleaning chemicals that my body was on toxic overload.

While the oils were the beginning of a life-long positive change in my health and wellness, they also dramatically changed my financial health.

First, I started using the oils to clean my home and care for my body, lowering my toxic exposure and load. Slowly, consistently with food, yoga, and lifestyle upgrades, I became stronger and more vibrant, regaining my health one day at a time. Learning how to clean my home with safer, natural, and non-toxic essential oils, I began to notice how my moods changed. Using Lemon and Peppermint essential oils actually brightened my mood even through mundane chores. Today, I use them to support my complete and optimal health.

As my health improved, my mind improved and all the dreams I had left behind once more became a possibility.

In 2007, I still suffered with pain and emotional swings occasionally, but I was getting stronger and more resilient. I was introduced to a more vigorous style of yoga, which opened my perspective to the possibility of optimal health. I could actually feel my body ease and release deep-seated stress and tension like opening a dam that had been blocking toxic release.

As my body grew stronger, my mind did as well. Using the oils to support the emotional upheaval created as long-held pain and tension melted away helped me continue toward optimal health.

All my life, I have wanted to help others feel better and be happy. Following a whole-food and Ayurvedic lifestyle, soon I became strong enough to follow my passion for sharing wellness with others. Because yoga proved to be a true healer, and as my relationship to my body improved, I began to treat it better, and my thoughts became healthier, I studied and trained to become a Yoga Teacher.

Shortly after, I felt so good that I even studied to become an Integrative Holistic Health Coach and Ayurveda Wellness Counselor so that I could empower my students and clients to achieve optimal health. Now, as an Essential Oil Educator, I teach people how to use oils to support their wellness.

Then, all this knowledge, all this training, all this passion for optimal wellness and all my courage was needed one Easter night. After the family festivities, my husband and I were having a great time preparing our dinner to the sounds of smooth mellow jazz. We were going to catch up on one of our favorite television shows while we ate. I walked upstairs, turned on the TV, and before I could sit down, I heard a loud banging on the counter.

I knew something was terribly wrong. I ran downstairs but before I reached the landing, I heard a large thump. At the bottom of the stairs, I turned the corner to see my husband lying on the kitchen floor convulsing, not breathing, hands drawn in and eyes bugged out. In an instant I had to make a decision: go to him, or call 911.

I reached in my purse for my phone and my oils. I knelt beside my husband, with one hand dialing 911 while the other hand opened a small bottle of Frankincense to calm both his stress and mine. I told the person on the phone that they needed to get there quick as I sprinkled him with Frankincense essential oil. You see, the love of my life, the boy who had taken me to prom and held my heart had started taking his last breaths. Harsh, mechanical inhales followed by long pauses, then an equally harsh mechanical exhales.

I put the phone down and I held him and I prayed. I stroked his forehead, inhaling the soothing aroma to ease my stress, then laid my hand on his heart.

He began to respond so I turned him on his side. There on the kitchen floor he was able to clear what had lodged in his throat. When the EMTs arrived, he had come around and had sat up against the cabinet. He told them he was dizzy and that his head hurt so they took him to the ambulance for a quick test. They told me he needed to go to the hospital to get his heart checked out. It was only because he kept complaining of head pain that an MRI was ordered. It revealed a large brain and spinal cord bleed. He was transported to a different hospital that could handle the neurological injury.

The first few hours I think he was in shock. He seemed aware and able to think. As the adrenaline wore off, his ability to think sequentially diminished and confusion set in.

The doctors and nurses were supportive but far from positive. They gave me their blessing to use my essential oils to help with emotional and immune support.

As his confusion dulled and his mental ability began to return, he was able to return to work a week after his fall. But there is side effect of traumatic brain injury that is silent and generally not spoken of—the emotional balance and stress resiliency. During his recovery, essential oils were a powerful tool to increase his emotional flexibility and stabilize his moods.

Looking back, I used a lot of citrus oils to support mood management for both of us. I cooked whole, organic, and super nutritious foods to support his body and brain to heal the way it is designed to do. I prayed prayers of thanksgiving for this man's life, blessings of abundant health, and patience to bear the changes that must happen in order for the body to heal.

Today my husband is healthy. He is by my side and supports me as I create a global wellness business. The same wonderful business that allowed me to take the necessary time to care for him as he recovered is the business I mentor my team to grow for themselves. I show them how to grow a sustainable, life-supporting business that gives them the freedom to shift focus toward life's unexpected priority shifts.

I use the oils in my home for everything from cleaning, to personal hygiene and skin care to supporting the systems in my body to function optimally. At my hot yoga studio, I use them to clean, for pest control, and to enhance stress resiliency for my students. I have also successfully created a thriving wellness-focused business and best of all, help my team to do the very same thing.

There was a time in my life when I had to give up everything, when I thought my life carried no value because of my illness. By the grace of God, that is no longer my story. I have restored my health and my belief in possibility and potential. Today, I am living the life of my dreams as I help others to experience their radiant optimal wellness and to achieve the financial peace and time freedom they desire.

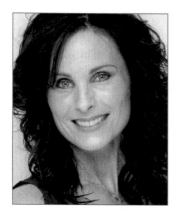

Rommy Kirby believes that you deserve to feel vibrant, healthy, and alive and that you can find your personal radiant optimal wellness. When asked what she does, she has a simple answer, "I help people feel better, manage their stress and have more energy so they can have more fun. What I teach is not rocket science. When I show you how to work with your body rather than against it, you become more resilient to stress, your weight balances, your energy and stamina increase, and life in general simply becomes more fun. It's not hard, but it does take effort. All change does." Married to the love of her life, the boy who took her to prom, Rommy lives just north of Nashville, where she owns a My HOT YOGA Place and Radiant Core Yoga School. She loves yoga, movement, and the peace of mind that comes with radiant health. Rommy Kirby holds an E-RYT, RYS, INHC, and AADP and is an Ayurveda practitioner. **Learn more: www.RommyKirby.com.**

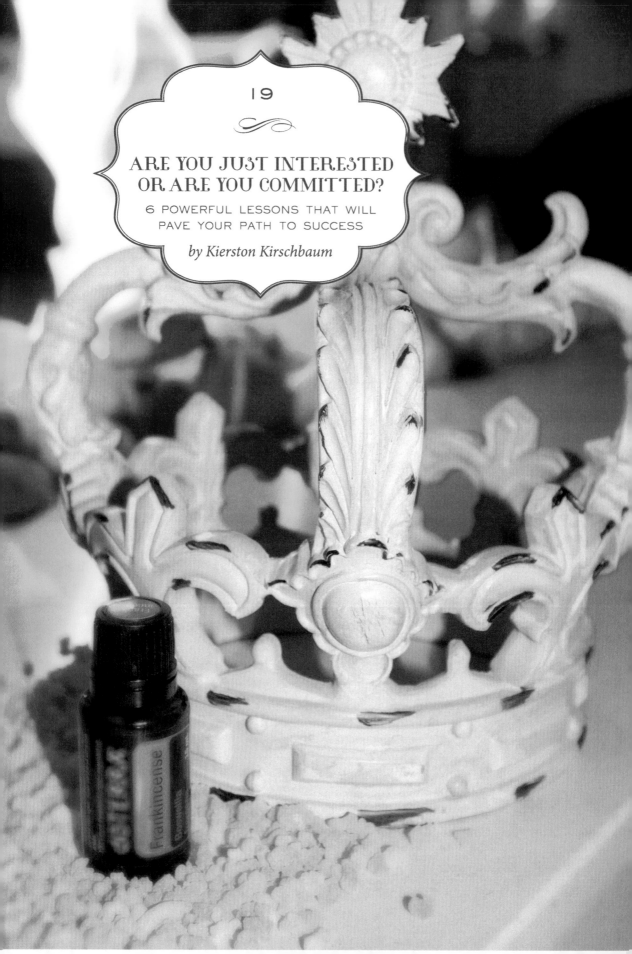

19

ARE YOU JUST INTERESTED OR ARE YOU COMMITTED?

6 POWERFUL LESSONS THAT WILL PAVE YOUR PATH TO SUCCESS

by Kierston Kirschbaum

So why do most people screw it up? Because the path has a toll—a price—and you have to answer it. That price comes in the form of a simple question:

Are you just interested or completely committed to living your dreams and goals?

Answering this question is not as easy as you think, but by the time you finish this short chapter you will gain the hidden insight you need through seven powerful lessons that will arm you with what you need on your road to success.

I once heard spiritual entrepreneur John Assaraf talk about the difference between interest and commitment. Interest in wealth or health or anything else doesn't mean that you'll do what it takes. But a person who is committed, Assaraf said, will succeed: "you'll learn what you need to learn, you'll rehearse what you need to rehearse, you'll practice, you'll drill, and you'll do everything that is needed to be done in order to achieve success."

I specifically remember a September day, more than three years ago. My newborn baby was screaming in my arms. Outside, leaves were falling and floating to the ground as my two-year-old son was playing with grandma's toys. We had just moved into my in-laws home, as we were desperately trying to save money and get back on our feet.

Feelings of despair, blame, and even hate looped uncontrollably in my mind. "Why couldn't we just rewind time?" Why couldn't go back to our old life?" Why did my husband make us move?" "Why did everything have to fall apart?" I resented everything that had thrust me into this new painful reality.

Just six months earlier, life was perfect—everything was planned to a "T." Financially, we were set, we were involved in our community and church, our kids had their best friends, and planning our next vacation was the top priority. Honestly, it couldn't get better, and we were very grateful.

But, I should have been known better. I wish God would have just knocked on my door and said, "Hey, Kierston, it's me. I just want to give you a heads up and let you know that the next couple years are, well, quite frankly they are going to be hard. But just be patient, have faith in me, be committed while I rearrange the pieces. Believe me, what I have in store will transcend your wildest dreams."

Lesson #1

When your life is being rearranged, when you are going through the hardest times in your life, you still have a choice. You may not be able to control your surroundings, but you can control you. You can decide to let it diminish your faith, overcome you, and take all control away, or you can fight with every last ounce of willpower to protect your faith in something greater, maybe even something better.

Just six months earlier the pieces started moving in our lives and I didn't even see it. Work started to crumble and my two young boys were experiencing some discomfort in their ears. We had been searching for a way to support their health naturally, but couldn't find any answers.

I could feel my heart tell me that there was another way. But what? I had no answers and it was eating at me.

The next day, a close friend called. "Remember that package of essential oils that you got at my house?" she said. "Well, you should try putting a little bit of Lavender and Basil around their ears. It should help ease their discomfort."

I jotted down the two names of the oils and promised my friend that I would try it. I was determined to help my sons; if Lavender and Basil could really support their health, I guess that's what I would do.

The next twenty-four hours transformed my life, not just because the two oils eased their discomfort and my sons were back to jumping off of their beds, but because I felt empowered. I don't even think that the word *empowered* can capture the feeling. Instead of feeling helpless, I now felt like I could do something.

I wondered how in the world I had never heard about essential oils, like it was some sort of conspiracy being kept from me. I remember lying in bed thinking of all of the other moms and friends who were dealing with the same hopeless feeling. I had to tell them.

Lesson #2

You can recognize your path to abundance, fulfillment, and purpose because when you first discover it, you feel like everything is possible—and it is. It's almost as if you are given a glimpse of the ending to keep you motivated to take the first step.

The next six months were a whirlwind of moving out of our home in Las Vegas, giving birth to our third baby boy, and figuring out what this passion for educating other moms about essential oils really meant.

It was on the eve of our departure from Las Vegas to Utah that one of the most critical moments took place in this incredible journey. We couldn't afford to rent a trailer, so we piled all of our stuff so high and in such an unorganized way that I thought we had hooked up the sleigh from *The Grinch Who Stole Christmas*. It was an embarrassing moment. Here we were in our beautiful neighborhood with our friends standing around, wondering why we couldn't afford to live there anymore, with our trailer and all of our stuff being held together with ropes.

But amongst all of the commotion and tears, a new friend walked into my house. This friend had been through similar hardships over the previous three years and had also found essential oils. She had experienced that same feeling of empowerment with her family and decided to build a business around her passion for empowering other moms. We were sitting in my empty living room and she looked at me dead in the eye and said, "Kierston, do what I tell you to do and I promise I will get you back in your home." Without hesitation I said, "I will, I will do whatever you tell me to do and I will get back here."

Lesson #3

Most people don't succeed just because of their God-given talents or abilities. They don't succeed because of a situation that arises where they have an opportunity to step up. Rather, most people succeed because someone believes in them when they don't believe in themselves, and they use that belief to propel themselves until they have a strong enough belief of their own.

Fast forward back to that fall day at my in-laws. I had regressed from a place of hope, inspiration, and desire to despair, blame, and regret. I would never return to my home. My friend's words seemed to fade from my mind and, with them, their power to inspire me.

Earlier that week she had challenged me to listen to an audio about positive affirmations and quotes from a man named Denis Waitley. I will never forget hearing his words as I drove down the road, "You have two primary choices in life. The first is to accept conditions as they exist, or the second is to take responsibility for changing them." Those words felt like someone had reached through the speakers and slapped me. Was I going to buy into the reasons why I couldn't succeed, like how I didn't have enough money to cover my monthly order or how I could fail? Or was I going to let today be the day that everything would change? That day would mark the day that all of those reasons why I *couldn't* would become the reasons why I *could*—why I *would* succeed.

Lesson #4

When you become committed, your reasons for being distracted—for blaming others, for believing the lies you tell yourself about failure and success—become the very fuel that drives the unquenchable thirst to succeed no matter what the odds may be.

Five months later, with the help of my best friend and upline leader, I barely qualified to attend Leadership Retreat in Park City, Utah. I like to call myself a "duct-tape Silver," because it didn't feel real. I even convinced my husband to come, even though he ended up taking care of our baby in the hall. I was the only person there from my upline's team—just she and I. I'm sure she was praying that something would sink in and add fuel to my fire. She had no idea what would happen next. (Or maybe she did!)

A beautiful mother at the Diamond level, who had recently finished Diamond Club, stood up to tell her story. In that moment—in that room of eight hundred people—my vision was opened up for a second and I could see the future. I told myself right then that I would do Diamond Club and hit Diamond. The following year I would speak on that same stage and tell my story.

Lesson #5

When you are committed to pursue your path, and can dispel all doubt and fear of failure, you then operate from a place where you will literally manifest what you want to accomplish. P.S.: MASSIVE ACTION is required.

Just as I had promised myself, I enrolled in Diamond Club, and I achieved Diamond in the last two months of the program. In fact, there was so much momentum that six months after hitting Diamond we hit Blue Diamond. I still remember looking down at my phone and reading "Emily Wright" on my caller ID. It was just thirty days before the next Leadership event was going to happen and I remember hearing her loving voice ask, "Would you speak at Leadership?"

Thirty days later I stood on that same stage and told my story of being the duct-taped Silver—how I had experienced a moment of clarity and an overwhelming sense that what was in store would surpass my wildest dreams. Two years from the day that my friend stood in my house and told me, "Do what I tell you to do and I will get back in your home," we moved back into our beautiful home. It was like a dream, but this time my husband was now working at home with me. We were spending every day together as a family, and we knew that we had found our path to greatness.

Our return marked a critical change in our motivation to succeed. It was now not about us but our responsibility to issue that same promise to all the people on our team.

Lesson #6

Motivation comes from many places. For some, it comes from material items and enjoying nice things. For others, it's about recognition and significance. But to live your life purpose and change the world, your motivation has to be rooted in your legacy—not how you improved your own life but how you impacted the lives of others and what that legacy was that you left in others.

Having been blessed with the ability to serve, teach, and lead people on this path is one of the greatest blessings we have been given. Sometimes we get asked, "When will you stop and be done?" Our answer to that is, "Never." Because the thrill of hearing people share their dreams and goals and helping them make that a reality through the power of essential oils is one of the most rewarding things in the world.

In the words of Jim Collins, "For, in the end, it is impossible to have a great life unless it is a meaningful life. And it is very difficult to have a meaningful life without meaningful work." We are blessed to have the most meaningful work in the world.

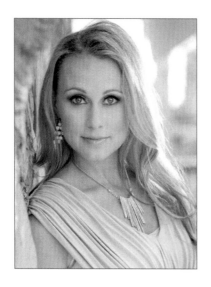

Kierston Kirschbaum is a mother, speaker, mentor, and creator of **EssentialOilExpert.com.** *She has created several popular training programs including Business Mastery and 6 Figure Health Heros. Kierston is an active member of her church and community, serving in volunteer positions in the young women's organization of her church, and as Mrs. Henderson America. She received her business degree at San Diego State University and has had her Real Estate license in California and Nevada, owned a mortgage company, and modeled for several clothing lines and magazines. She is the proud mother of four amazing boys and enjoys traveling the world with them and her husband, Kyle. Kierston's passion has always been to help mothers be empowered to take control of their families' health and wealth. In just three years, she founded a huge team of Essential Oil Experts that now spans the globe. She enjoys teaching others how to create the life of their dreams and leading the way for many women to follow!* **Learn more: www.claimpurepower.com; Kierston@essentialoilexpert.com.**

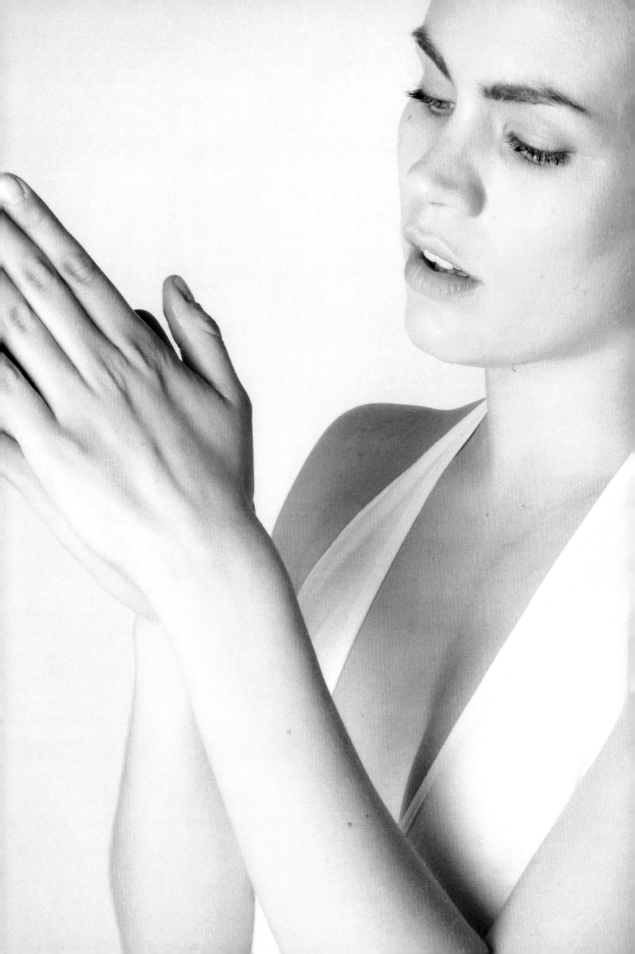

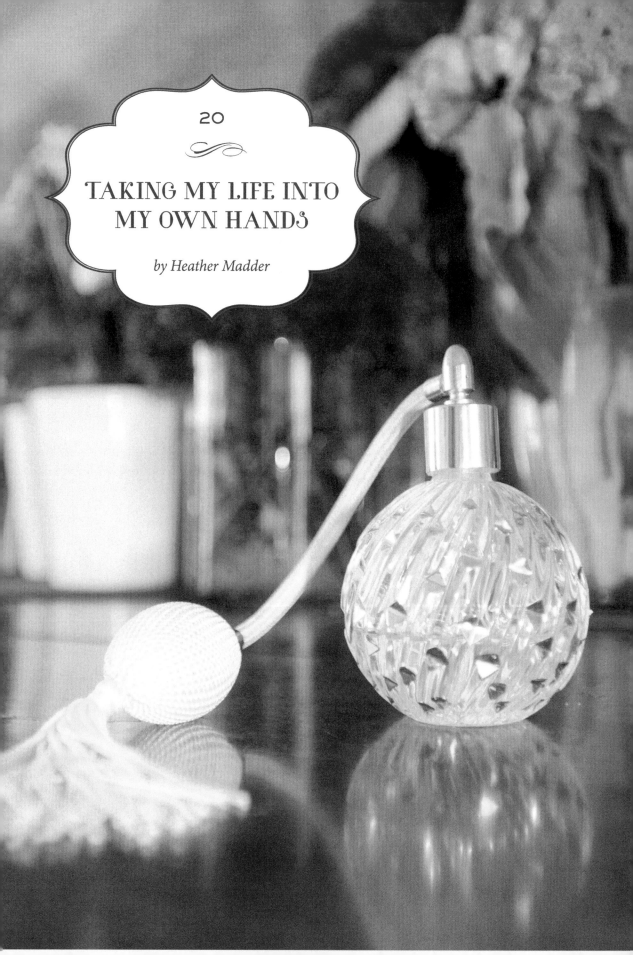

20

TAKING MY LIFE INTO MY OWN HANDS

by Heather Madder

"IF YOU TELL ANYONE, I'LL KILL YOU," HE WARNED, HIS FINGERS AROUND MY THROAT.

As he stood up, I could still feel his fingers around my neck. I turned my head to the side and lay there quietly while I waited for him to leave. He slipped on his shoes and addressed me one more time before he departed. "Remember what I said," he commanded. I stared at the sagebrush in the distance, avoiding his face, and nodded. He disappeared. I lay in the dirt, shaky and frozen.

I closed my eyes. I knew I had to get up, but my body was searing in pain and wouldn't move. I took in a long, deep breath through my nose, still flat on the dry summer earth. Motionless, I stared at the blue sky brushed with a few white, wispy clouds. My legs were heavy and lead-like. My heart was still pounding and felt like a hard fist was banging on my chest, my face damp with tears.

I knew I couldn't stay here. I drew in another long breath. And this time, I rolled over onto my side and then to my forearms and rested my body on my hands and knees, my face low to the dusty ground, my body in a folded praying position.

After a few more moments, I pushed my weight onto my legs and stood up. I slowly got dressed, and then stumbled my way back to the house. As I walked, I came to my senses and remembered what to do.

I would find the group. I would join them and pretend I had lost something and had been looking for it. I would act as though nothing was wrong—again. I believed the threats—that I would die if I spoke of it, so I shoved this experience—and the other experiences like it, in a vault away from the world, away from my ability to put words to it, and away from everyone's view, including my own conscious remembrance.

I was nine.

In my mid-thirties, I began to have nightmares and other symptoms. I had no explanation for my feelings of constant panic, or the paralyzing fear I felt if someone walked up too quickly behind me or unexpectedly rang my doorbell.

I also happened to be a weekly church-going mom of four, married to a hard-working husband of fifteen years. I had a blossoming career as an author and talk radio show host and had a coaching business. I helped people think positively and find meaning in their lives, and there was a brilliant, inspiring, and tenacious side to who I was.

I had been blessed in many ways, and yet life felt inexplicably arduous to me. Most mornings, I would lay in bed awake staring at the ceiling waiting for my arms and legs to gain enough life and for my heart to wrap around its desire to fight another day. When I was ready, I would make my way down the stairs, and as I descended into my life, my happy face would pull itself again over my real face, like a virtual mask. I wore it for everyone—my husband, children, friends, clients, church members—everyone got the "happy face."

I made that life work by tapping into my talent and tenacity. But I had not yet developed the language, or even the kindness to myself, to share what I was privately experiencing.

I had often feared that terrible things had happened to me early in life, and my nightmares indicated this might be so. But my conscious memories were vaulted deeply enough that I couldn't recall the actual events. I stayed in the denial (and numbness) of forgetting while also trapped in the pain.

In my late thirties, my painful symptoms increased and I began to pray for answers and speak to the people close to me about what I was going through. Over time, God prepared my tender mind for the truth, and eventually He allowed those memories to return to me. For twenty-one months, like rats scurrying from under the door, memories darted forward. With each memory, the sights, sounds, and terror of the moment would rise up from its hiding place and make its way through my system. One minute I would be doing the dishes, and the next, I would be swallowed by intense fear.

After months of this it became obvious to me and the professionals I was working with that I had been suffering from side effects of violent physical and sexual abuse. As I understood the reason for my symptoms, I sought for answers and visited more than twenty-five different professionals. In time, those memories and their dark contents left my system and I experienced profound peace and love. Sometimes, that love was so intense, I felt enveloped by it completely.

During this season, I reached daily for the support of essential oils.

The first thing the oils did for me was help me regain a sense of control. Because life had felt beyond my control for so long, it was such a relief to be able to administer them to myself; the ability to feel better was in my own hands. The scent of Basil or Lavender would make me breathe easier or feel calmer. White Fir on the bottom of my feet made me feel grounded. It wasn't just the oil itself but the act of applying it myself that empowered me and allowed me to regain a sense of control over my feeling good again. I found that the oils supported me physically and emotionally through this difficult time. I felt like I was wading through hell to get to heaven. This was no small journey, and the sheer magnitude of this transition was exhausting to me in every way.

I wanted to be able to take care of myself and my children and continue on with my career as much as I was capable of doing, and I honestly don't believe I would have been able to do it at the same capacity without using them regularly. Citrus Bliss® and Lime diffusing in my kitchen is a favorite way to start my morning, the uplifting aroma of those oils awakening my mind and heart and reminding me to stay in the present and make the best of the day ahead. For an immunity boost while traveling, I use On Guard, and to lift my mood for public speaking, I used Elevation. I remember one particular event, I was sitting in the audience waiting for my turn to go on stage and my body was lifeless in the chair. I shook Elevation onto my hands and forearms (it was way too much!) and it suddenly energized me just before it was my turn. I spoke with passion and excitement, and many of those people became my clients and have since joined my team.

Most importantly, the oils were helping me to feel peaceful about what happened in the past. For example, my father had been one of my abusers and had died of a drug overdose before we had the opportunity to mend our relationship. At first, I felt disadvantaged and angry. Death made things so final and I felt I had lost something that could never be regained. I felt particularly drawn to Frankincense, and when I read about it, I understood why. Frankincense is an oil that connects us to our Divine Father and helps us feel loved and supported. I realized that even though my earthly father had died, I had a Heavenly Father whose love and care for me was constant and was something I could draw on in the present time. I really feel that Frankincense aided my ability to connect to that reality, and today my life is so overflowing with love that emptiness seems very far away.

Today, I live a healthy, beautiful, active life that I absolutely love. My husband David and I have four children who astound us with their brightness and brilliance. I speak to people all over the world about truth and wholeness, and I also lead a large team as a Blue Diamond with dōTERRA.

My life story isn't a sad one. For me, it's a profound journey of self-discovery! It provided me with unique advantages and powerful insight that will always remain with me. In the face of piercing lies of personal devaluement, I learned the truth of who I really am, and I have cemented that knowledge in an unforgettable way. As low as my insecurity once was, my self-certainty has grown much higher. I love myself completely—without exception—and nothing can separate me from that. I have no fear of pain or death, because I know the path of peace and deliverance. I have learned how to speak truth boldly and to create happiness on my own terms, without apology. Through the darkness, I found God, and that is my most precious relationship.

When I was young, I always wanted someone to save me from what was happening—I wanted someone to rescue me and take me away from the madness. When I grew up (especially emotionally), I realized that no one was coming. And *that* saved me.

No one was going to get my body off the ground. No one was going to make me move forward. No one was going to force me to love myself. No one was going to help me believe in who I was. No one was going to repair—or even apologize—for what happened. No one was going to make everything all better.

I had to do that for myself now—I was the one I had been waiting for. And after that, I saw I needed God just as much. When I realized that, my whole life changed. Every prison we are in has a door and it unlocks from the inside. I made a firm choice to take healing into my own hands and never stop until it was complete. I have made that decision over and over again every day for many years now and taking accountability for my own wholeness, and not blaming others, gave me the power and motivation to do it.

I chose to partner with God every step of the way, because He is my Creator. He loves me deeply and infinitely and has infused His name into every one of my cells. He told me to ask Him for help, and I did. As often as I asked, He showed me the steps and helped me to have the courage to take each one.

I am especially thankful for essential oils, because they have been my most consistent, most used healing tool. I know that the earth that has been created to house the human race also has the intelligence to support us while we are here. As I have used those gifts, I have seen my body and mind increase in strength and will forever be grateful for the journey that allowed me to have the knowledge I have today.

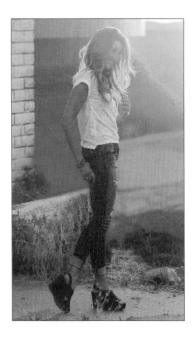

Heather Madder *is the mother of four and married to her soulmate, David. She's an author, coach, and dōTERRA Blue Diamond. Her personal mission is to help create a world where people are free from limitations, living from their highest selves, and where peace, love, consciousness, prosperity, and joy are an everyday state of being.* **Learn more: www.HeatherMadder.com; admin@heathermadder.com.**

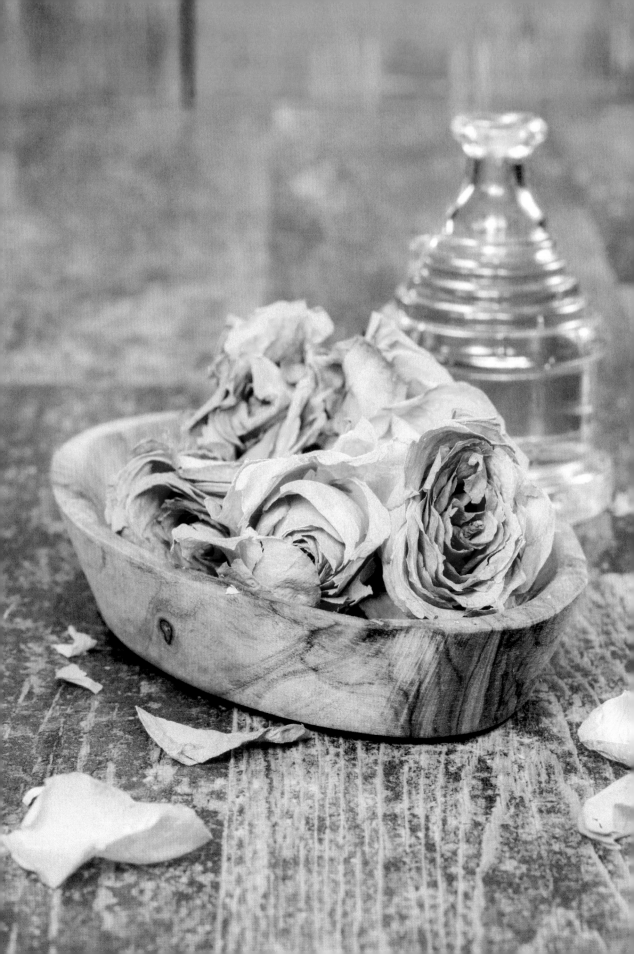

THOUGHTS ON
LEADERSHIP

by Heather Madder

A business can only be as healthy as the people who run it. Energize and rejuvenate your mind, body, and soul every day and never miss. Because your business is built from the inside out, what you create from stress or emotional deficit will become problematic in one way or another down the road. When you are happy and healthy, that energy calls out to other happy and healthy people and gives life to everything you touch. Your first priority is taking the best care of your own inner space, and from that place, you will build a life and business that is strong and beautiful.

A great business is built by doing the most important things that create the greatest results. You don't need to be crazy-busy, exhausted, and overwhelmed to get what you want. Just be wise and disciplined! Ask yourself: What are the most effective actions that get me where I want to go? Do those things first when you are at your highest energy, and plan to do them over and over again every month. Say no or "not right now" (without an apology) to everything else. You owe it to yourself and your family to create success on these terms. In the end, a happy, peaceful life is one of the greatest gifts you can give the planet, and everyone has equal power to create this for themselves.

Never compare yourself to another person. Comparison is a poison that sucks the life out of everything you do. You are good enough just as you are, right now, this moment. When you really take that in and you feel it, everything in your life will emerge with beauty and perfection. Doors will throw themselves wide open. People will flock to you because the whole world responds to people who love themselves. This is what we all want the most, and when you give that to yourself, you will be a light of positive change wherever you go. Self-love is not something you can earn; it is something that you *choose*.

Be your own biggest cheerleader. There is only one person you have ever needed to believe in you—and that's you. By the time you wonder, "What do they think of me?" you have already betrayed yourself. What do *you* think of you? That's what matters. What we want the most is to believe in ourselves as we follow the path that is right for us and create happiness on our own terms.

Don't stress about the future. Address one day at a time. Trust that life is taking care of you and that your own perfect plan is unfolding. The more you trust, the more peaceful you will be and the faster you will travel. Seek for divine inspiration and ask, "What is my next step?" Listen and just do that. It takes 58,000 steps to climb Mount Everest, but how is that great feat achieved? By taking one step, and then another. You only have one thing to do at a time. Bring your focus and attention in the here and now and live this day as fully as you can. When you see the view from the top of the mountain you will see how perfect your life plan has been and how much you have achieved, and you will know that life had your back the whole time.

Effective leaders focus on the right things and they stay calm and clear-minded. They don't get pulled into drama and they don't become reactive. As a leader, you will be faced with countless situations that challenge you. In resolving conflict, listen intently to every side, but always stay neutral. Don't react.

Take the time you need to separate what is important from what is not important and make your decisions based on the highest principles of integrity that will create long-term well-being. You are not here to please everyone. There will always be a certain percentage of people who are not pleased by you, and that's a sign things are perfectly in order. You are here to lead with truth and clarity, so keep your focus on what really matters.

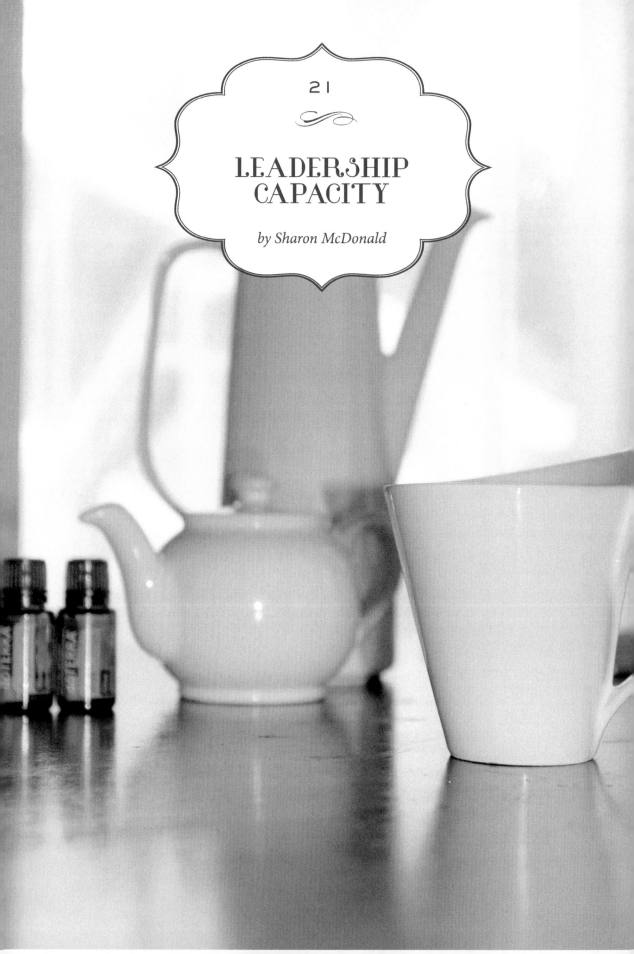

21

LEADERSHIP CAPACITY

by Sharon McDonald

ESSENTIAL OILS AND NUTRITION GRABBED MY ATTENTION EARLY ON IN MOTHER-HOOD BECAUSE I WAS LOOKING FOR HOPE IN MY CHAOS AND A CHANCE TO BE MY FAMILY'S FIRST DEFENSE.

My first big exposure to a world of natural health and wellness solutions happened when we were moving home from Europe, where we had lived for five years. There, we walked everywhere; we ate delicious, organic, fresh foods; we had plenty of options for great education, sports, and natural wellness; and we were successful in bringing leadership to our community. It was ideal!

But then, just two weeks before moving back to the United States in June 2007, I broke the fifth-metatarsal on my left foot. Our home was getting packed in two days, we were going through Washington, D.C. on our way home to show our children their American heritage, and I was in a cast and using crutches. I would not be partying it up before we left; neither would I be packing, cleaning, walking, running, or preparing our new home and new life on my own. I had to—quite literally—lean on others. This is when I began to learn that we never do it alone! People come into our lives all the time to guide the way, help us create spaces, make memories, and lead the way to success. We cross the finish line—or don't—but along the way we have crowds of people in front, in back, and on the sidelines rooting for us. There is a lot of power in that. Wearing a cast, I saw others in front and in back of me, and on the sidelines serving and loving me, as they gave back to our family the way we had given to so many.

A dear friend had recently been introduced to essential oils and was super excited to share the power of nature's botanicals. I was skeptical and thought it was a placebo. Besides, I had always said no to network marketing. But then, more than three months after the break, my bone was still not knitting—the report was the same: zilch, nada, zip! So I tried what my friend recommended: Birch and Helichrysum. And a month later I was walking around.

My question was, if these crazy oils could support my body in this powerful way, what else could they do? We successfully used Peppermint essential oil for just about everything after our initial introduction, yet, that is as far as it went. Essential oils worked for us. However, I began to see how I was my becoming my family's first defense in nutrition and healthy options and desired to be that "one" for someone else. It was very empowering, almost addictive, we are forever grateful that Jodi chose to be the one by opening her mouth and offering another solution in a time of need. Because of her.... I said yes! Because I said yes, I have been the "one" for many, many others. There is much gratitude in my heart for the "crock of voodoo in a bottle" offered to me. No placebo, no voodoo, just sustainable solutions that allow us to be the "one" defense in our home for our family and our community that we can count on.

All this prepared me for when one of our children started having sensitivities to new situations. That summer, I was invited to experience essential oils. I was inspired by the crisp quality and power I felt from their purity. I told my husband that though we had spent $400 with a different company just three months earlier, this was the "real deal." In reply, he told me to go all in: "I think you should do this as a business." Our oldest was thirteen and the youngest just two. Life was crazy, messy, and very full. But after a month of mulling it over and pondering the potential outcomes, I decided to run with it. The goal? To gather as many people as we could to the finish line so we could all get back to our daily routines and celebrate our victories along the way. What actually happened had greater purpose in changing our lives forever.

Life happened to each of our business partners. Some of these people lost their homes, a spouse, jobs, hope, marriages, and health. Some were "all in"; while others were finding where the business fit into their purpose. Our team grew in strength, experiences, and success. And then tragedy struck much closer to home. A year into our oils journey and achieving the rank of Diamond, we lost my dear sweet father to lung cancer. The day of his funeral, we miscarried our sixth child and my health began to decline. Three years after signing on, we achieve Blue Diamond, representing less than 1 percent of the company. But, around that same time, I received a pathology report that rocked our world, and a week later I was hospitalized for blood clots in both lungs. Life had changed.

I believe that what we do with negative circumstances is what matters. We rolled with it and transformed our game plan to gather our team close and let them cheer us on for a season. As a family, we decided that I would not teach at nights or on the weekends for a year to gather my strength, heal, and regroup. However, I did not stop living. Everyone rallied around from the sidelines, from behind and in front to keep me on my course. Was it easy? No! Was it what I wanted? No! Was it needed? Yes! I learned through that process to *listen*. I learned that life is not a race, and healing comes in ways we never imagine.

If we listen, our intuition tells us where to go, what to do, and where to find light. If we listen, we are able to lift others, to serve them, and to raise them to their highest potential and our needs are met completely. Each of us had the drive to chart our own path, lead our own lives, and show others how find freedom with our healing hands. Transformation offers a new voice that will come with power and drown out the battles we can find ourselves involved with, if we slow down and let go. When we see others not moving forward, do we judge? Or do we lift and share our light? Remember, this could be the hardest battle they have ever fought. They may be trying to "roll with it" and manifest something new. Besides, life isn't fair. But you can be. Are you willing to share your light and healing hands?

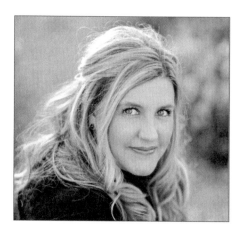

*Sharon McDonald is a thriver, gypsy at heart, entrepreneur, lover of people, veteran teacher and curriculum designer, and a sassy mama of five! Her father reminded her often she had a purpose from the time she could walk and she has been sharing that purpose ever since. Currently, she is the head Chaos Coordinator at The Farm. **Learn more: www.gogreenessentials.com; gogreenessentials@gmail.com.***

THOUGHTS ON
LEADERSHIP

by Sharon McDonald

The capacity we have to lead is determined by our desires to strengthen those around us. When we love ourselves, our families, our friends, our neighbors, and those we serve, we find meaning in what we do. When we offer our healing hands, we lead our lives in a way that brings peace, hope, and prosperity.

Life has its way, and circum-stances can certainly be overwhelming at times. I have come to learn three things that lead people to success regardless of what comes their way. I have lived these principles and believe them to be true:

What we do with negative circumstances is what really matters.

If we roll with it, we can transform ourselves to greater capacity. When life gets messy, what do we do?

React, or act?

Bury our head, or look up?

Give in and become a victim?

Or do we rise up to chart a course and become the victor?

We never are alone. There is always a team of people behind us, ahead of us and on the sidelines rooting for our success.

Life has a way of helping us learn our capacity to go the distance regardless of what may come our way. It seems to me that success comes from the hard knocks of life, yet the important thing is how we respond to those challenges, to the momentum, to the honor, and to the disappointments.

Want good grades? Study hard. Want to make the team? Practice hard. Want to be healthy? Eat right and exercise consistently. Want to accompany the choir? Practice hours and hours to be prepared enough to see success. Want that job? Go get it, or create an income with fresh ideas and a great campaign that attracts it. Want a leadership position? Present yourself as an ambassador of people and gain their trust. Want life to be "fair"? Sorry to say *mon frere*, life is not fair. A fair is a county competition where we compete to show our animals, ride rides, eat obscene amounts of greasy foods, play games, and watch the rodeo and parade while eating cotton candy. Life is not fair.

Life can be messy, and is not free from bias, dishonesty, or injustice! Storms come, failures happen, 5 extra pounds can turn into 10 when we're not paying attention, illness can shatter hope, people are fickle, children disobey, lives are taken early, loved ones pass away, and success can be just on the other side of disappointment if we will be patient in our suffering. What matters is how we find meaning in the mess, which offers hope to others seeking healing hands to lift them and light to show the way. This is where the value lays.

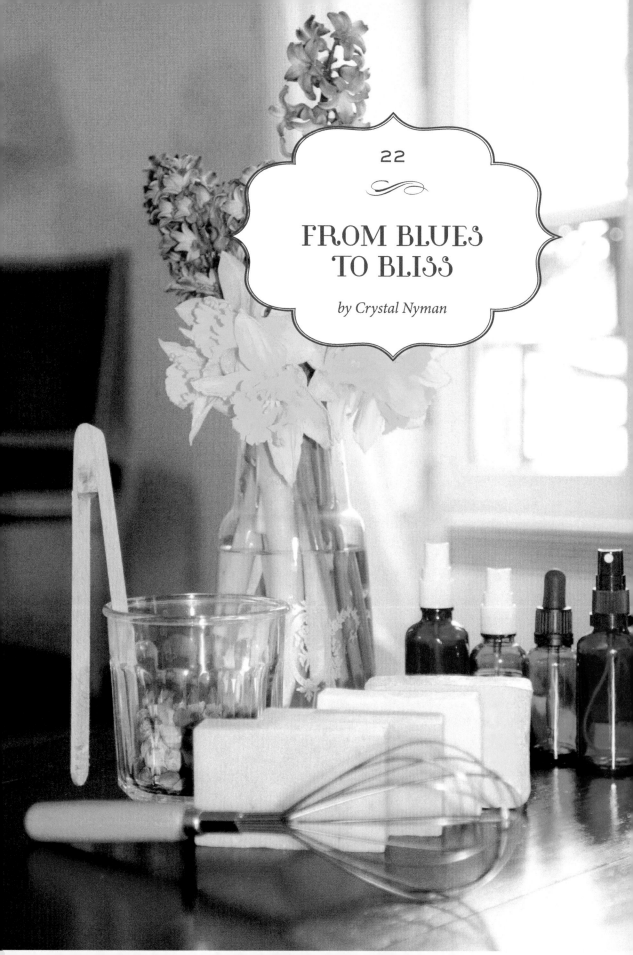

22

FROM BLUES TO BLISS

by Crystal Nyman

Other girls may dream of having kids and being a mom or having a career. I wanted all of it! I wanted that handsome prince who would treat me as a princess. I wanted children of my own who I could love and care for. I dreamed about being a confident career woman who made a difference in others' lives. You see, I love people! I love hearing their stories and problems. I love trying to figure out why people behave the way they do and think the way they think. I love guiding them to find solutions and empowering them to create the life they dream of—to go from a state of blues to a life of bliss!

At eighteen I felt like going to one year of college was long enough to decide it was time to get married. I thought I had found my prince who I would be with forever. Some marriages work out even when they start out so young. Not mine. Seven years later, I ended up divorced. My life was shattered! I had no idea what to do or where to go. What did this mean about me? Where was my "happily ever after" I thought happens once you are married? It played on every emotion possible. How would I provide for my three-year-old son? I was so afraid of the unknown. Little did I know it was just the beginning of a long roller-coaster ride.

I struggled to feel like myself. I got to where I didn't want to eat at all because everything affected my gut except chocolate chips and almonds. My mom showed up at my house one day with a bag of vitamins and supplements and told me I needed to take these as I was getting way too thin. I realized then I needed more nutrition. I tried my best to take in what I could stand to eat. I wanted to be healthy, but I just didn't know where to find the answers! I began looking for solutions.

Just two and half years later I remarried. I thought it would be much better this time, especially since I met my soon-to-be husband at church. Boy was I wrong! The next five and a half years were the most difficult of my life. We struggled to make ends meet. Near the end of our marriage, he was hospitalized for a week and we had no health insurance. We had more debt than we could keep up with, and it weighed on us so heavily that we eventually had to file bankruptcy. I had never in my life been at such a low point even though I had many low points. It was the worst suffocating feeling to not know how you're going to pay for food, rent, car, or electricity. I felt like such a failure!

As I was working four different commission-type jobs, I was approached by a co-worker asking me to come check out a "business opportunity" with an essential oils company. "No way!" I told him. I already had way too much on my plate and hardly had any time to spend with my son. Why would I even think to look at another job? With a little persuasion he got me to come to a free dinner. Days later I attended an annual convention to learn more. I couldn't help but wonder what I was doing there and why they talked about how these essential oils were changing lives. It sounded crazy. The next week I bought a kit with a variety of oils in it. I immediately started to use them for my son. He loved how they made him feel. I knew I'd better learn more. I went to classes and learned other ways to use the essential oils and why they worked. It all started to make sense.

Then I started to use them for myself. Holy moly! They helped me so much I thought, "Where the heck have these been for the last several years of my life?" I loved what they were doing for myself, for my son, and for my loved ones. I started a new journey from that point on. I was skeptical that this could ever be something that would become successful as a business but decided I would give it a shot for ninety days and treat it like a real job. If after the ninety days it wasn't progressing then I was going to quit everything I was doing and go get a single job so I could have the time I needed and wanted with my son. For that trial period, I quit the other jobs and focused on just sharing the oils with others.

To my surprise, after ninety days my business was continuing to grow, slowly but surely. I'll never forget having the opportunity to sit with Dave Stirling, founding executive and CEO of dōTERRA, about the same time. He said to me with such confidence, "Crystal, in just a few months you will be making a very good income." I thought again to myself that he was crazy! He assured me that it didn't matter that I didn't believe it yet but that I could rely on his faith. I so desperately hoped and prayed with all of my heart he would be right.

Just four months into my oils business, my second marriage ended. I was confident that sometimes there are better things in store for us even when at the moment we can't see it. What I did know is that I would be okay and so would my son because I had done this before, and I knew I could do it again.

I pressed forward on my journey with amazing support from my team leaders. They would not let me fail! They kept me going when things got tough and I wasn't sure if it would work. Things continued to progress each month, and little by little I realized I was being greatly blessed with a residual income I couldn't even begin to replace with another job.

Dave Stirling was right! I was starting to make the money he assured me I would. I was ecstatic! The best part about it was that I could provide for my son and myself by simply helping others learn how to incorporate natural products in their own home for their health and wellness. I got to listen to people's problems and help guide them to find solutions. I got to have the flexibility to set my own schedule so I could be the kind of mom I wanted to be. I got to show others how they could also create the financial freedom they were looking for. My life was better than ever before! I had gone from blues to bliss. The only thing missing at this point was my prince.

As all fairytales would have it, I have found my happily ever after! I am now married to my handsome prince I dreamed of who treats me as the most beautiful princess. I am blessed with children I always wanted and a thriving business where I get to really help others find natural solutions. In turn, it blesses our family with a monthly income ten times the amount Dave told me would happen and continues to grow. Wow! I would have never thought this could happen to me.

During life's challenges, it can be hard to see the light at the end of the tunnel. But when you keep going and never give up, you will get to that light. And it is worth every tear that was shed along the way to know such extreme joy! From blues to bliss… you can get there too.

Crystal Nyman worked as a mortgage loan officer for more than sixteen years. Although business comes naturally for her, Crystal's passion is helping others. Raised with the philosophy that holistic and natural remedies are sought first, Crystal has a diverse background in health and wellness. She completed her personal training certification in 2003, yet was seeking to understand the deeper wisdom of healing through mind-body connection, which led her to the Journey Practitioner's Program. She received her certification in 2007 for Journey therapy, an alternative healing modality. She guides her clients on a journey of healing emotionally, physically, mentally, and spiritually. Crystal was introduced to dōTERRA in 2009. Having had prior expe- 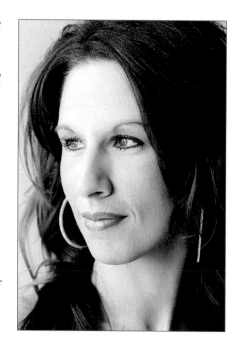 *rience in other network marketing companies, this one stood out to her as unique. She feels that essential oils were a return to the wisdom of the ancients. Crystal has since become one of dōTERRA's top leaders, instilling others with the confidence that they too can live a life from blues to bliss. Crystal resides in Kaysville, Utah, with her husband Jeff and their four kids. She enjoys travel, outdoor adventure, music, and golf. Learn more: frombluestobliss@gmail.com.*

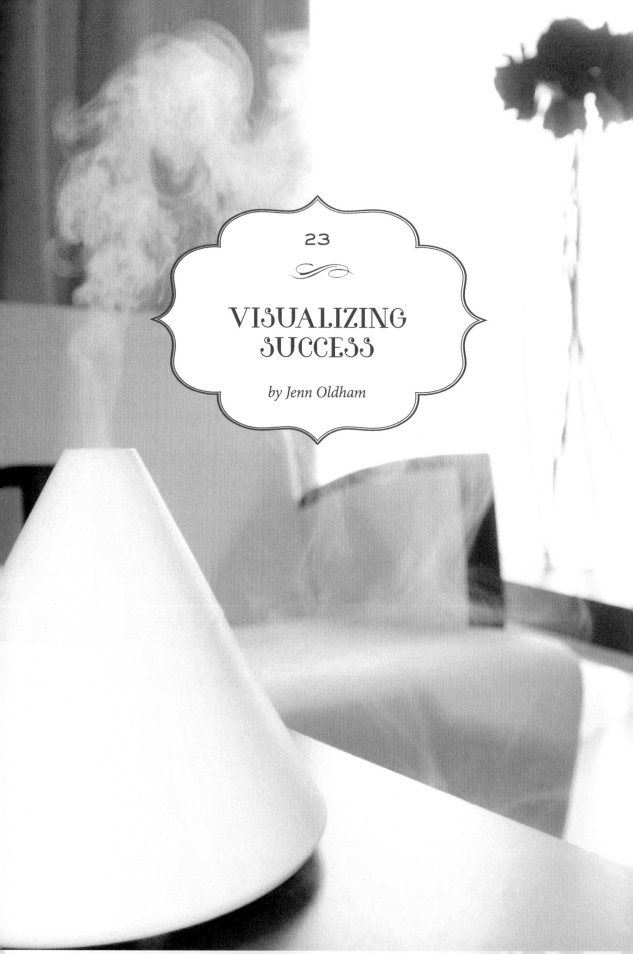

23

VISUALIZING SUCCESS

by Jenn Oldham

That didn't mean I was willing to get involved in the business. I was not going to get behind taking advantage of my friends and family. Also, I wanted to be a mom and didn't want something that would take my attention away from my daughter.

Then, as I saw how powerful the oils were, I wanted other moms to experience the same things. I had to tell people! And so I tested the waters with the business. But I held back because I didn't want to take time away from my most important priority—my daughter.

My husband and I were struggling financially, and we rarely had the money to do what we wanted and needed to do. It really started to hit home that an essential oils business could literally change our lives. As I became more serious about the business, it wasn't long before my income from sharing the oils was making our house payment. I couldn't believe what doors were being opened to us because we were making ends meet! So I set my sights on a life-changing income.

Life hit another snag when, in the fall of 2011, I found myself facing infertility. If I wanted more children—and I did!—I would need to have them through in vitro fertilization (IVF), which would cost about $13,000. It was a staggering expense. But with our goal in mind, I decided yet again to step it up a notch and really crank it out with my oils business.

By November, I was pregnant with a set of twins. Wow! I wanted to be pregnant, but the idea of twins was a little overwhelming, especially alongside my plans with my business. Two months later I achieved the rank of "duct tape Gold." I slipped back to Silver for a couple of months before moving forward again.

In March 2012, I was fully committed to hitting Diamond by June, the month I was anticipating my twins. I was missing an entire fourth leg, and I also had several other gaps in two of my three existing legs. But I was determined.

After declaring my intentions for reaching the rank of Diamond by that June, I bought a massive whiteboard. There, I drew my organization on the board and visualized what needed to happen over the next three months. At first it was a little depressing because I realized how far I had to go. Then, I realized that if I was going to hit the rank I wanted, I needed to stay committed, be proactive, and know where I was going. With my team visualized on the board, I knew exactly where I needed volume. Having those empty holes where volume needed to be helped me to be creative with how I could get the spots filled. Every day I set my intentions on how to fill those gaps. I worked very closely with my frontline leaders, and we worked hard to make success happen.

I collaborated at least once a week with each of my leaders, and we made a game plan for that week so that we could see what needed to be done. We just went through the basics of sharing, inviting, hosting, and enrolling. Keeping it simple helped my business grow the fastest. The simpler I kept it, the more people who wanted to join along with me.

Each month that went by, I was closer and closer to my goal and I was so excited that it was going to happen. And then June rolled around and I was on bedrest. I wasn't sure how to make it happen, but I was determined! I wasn't going to give up. Sure, I wasn't able to teach classes the conventional way, but that didn't stop me from teaching online or teaching sitting on someone's couch. I did it several times with great success.

My point is, when you set your mind to something, map it out, and look at your goals every day, you figure out ways to make it happen. Hitting Diamond is 100 percent a decision, not something that you just get lucky with. You have to decide that it is truly what you want and go for it. You need to really have a hunger for it.

I'm not an advocate of giving up everything for the goal that you want. Boundaries are crucial, and you must be willing to take care of yourself. You are your biggest asset and you don't want to mistreat it! You want to last for a long time. I definitely had goals and I pushed hard, but I also knew what I was not willing to do. For example, I was not willing to teach a class if it required standing, jumping, or moving; I wasn't putting my babies at risk. But if I could teach while following doctor's orders, I was more than happy! That is an example of boundaries I set. It may seem silly and something that you should already know, but success is a mindset! You must decide that you are in it to win.

June kept barreling along, and it did not look like I was going to hit my goal of Diamond. But I didn't let negative thoughts keep me from succeeding. As the month was coming to a close and I was several thousand away from my goal, I was absolutely determined to figure out a way and... I did! I am convinced that I achieved my goal because I set my sights on it and didn't give up. Hard work, determination, and perseverance are a great recipe for miracles to unfold.

By the last day of the month in June 2012, I was officially a Diamond. It was so surreal! It was so fun to achieve a rank that required so much. However, I had my sights on great success and even bigger achievements.

I learned a lot that following year about how to make a business work and excel without going completely crazy. I set very firm office hours, blocked out time, and stuck to a schedule. I hired a coach who helped me figure out what I needed to do to become successful, and I learned how to really lead and influence a team.

In October 2013, I reached the rank of Blue Diamond. It took me longer than it would have, and sometimes I struggled with trusting my ability to lead and influence others. But I was leading! I had several thousand people looking to me for leadership. I had fabulous leaders who were doing great things, but I couldn't put my goals on their shoulders and expect them to make my dreams come true. I had to create success. The biggest lesson that I learned between the rank of Diamond and Blue Diamond is that my success was in my hands and up to me, no matter how many people were on my team.

Over the past year, I've learned that I can create the culture of empowerment that I want on my team. It is a great feeling to know that so many lives have been changed because I decided to take a chance on myself and build a business. I am so grateful for the woman who introduced me to dōTERRA. This business is about believing in yourself and your abilities, being determined, and being willing to figure out how to make it work.

Enjoy the journey! It's a very worthwhile one that will teach you many lessons along the way. I love essential oils and hope you will allow them to bless your life as much as they have blessed my life.

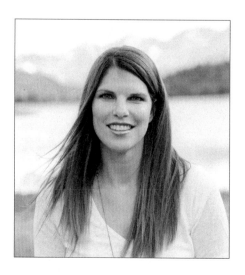

*When **Richard and Jennifer Oldham** were first introduced to dōTERRA by Roger and Teresa Harding, essential oils were very foreign to their way of living. But Jennifer felt like they should give it a chance. She explained, "I convinced Richard that we should at least enroll to see how we liked the oils. Together, we discovered that dōTERRA was a completely unique company in the network marketing industry, and we fell in love! We slowly evolved into the business builders that we are."*

*Jennifer and Richard are committed to not simply accepting excuses but to creating results. They have not let any excuse hold them back from achieving great goals. Jennifer feels that her biggest accomplishment was when they continued to achieve the rank of Diamond with newborn twins and an active three-year-old. "I had every excuse in the book to not succeed," she said. "But it was so important for me to achieve my goals that I made it happen. I was only willing to accept results. I do not feel that I am a hero but just an example of achieving success regardless of circumstances." With this positive outlook and a drive to make things happen, the Oldhams are sure to continue blazing through difficult times to achieve great things. **Learn more: www.EOBuilder.com.***

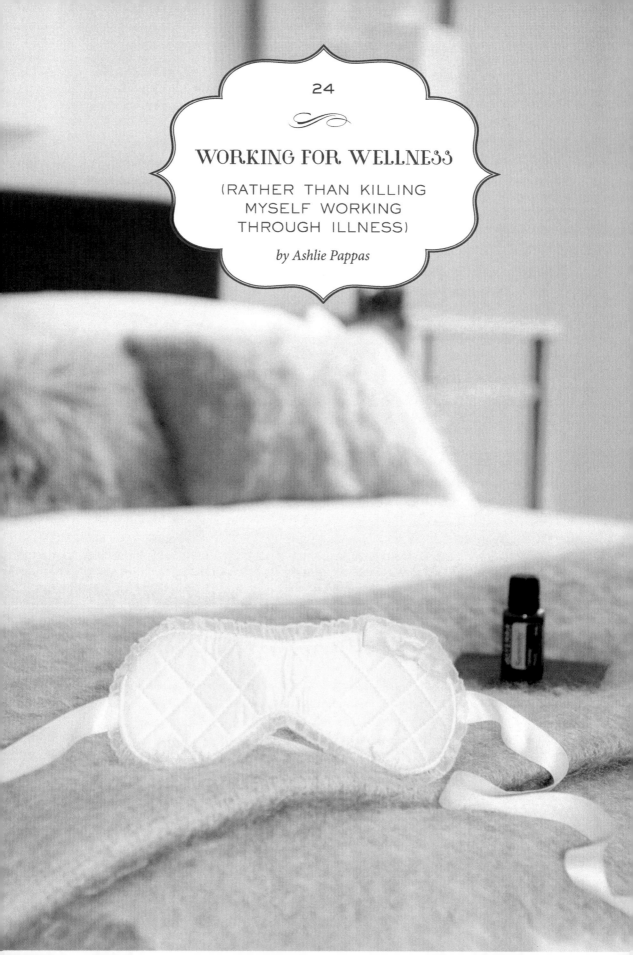

24

WORKING FOR WELLNESS

(RATHER THAN KILLING MYSELF WORKING THROUGH ILLNESS)

by Ashlie Pappas

I BEGAN MY "ADULT" LIFE A LITTLE LATE IN THE GAME. AFTER HIGH SCHOOL I WANTED TO TAKE A YEAR OFF TO "EXPERIENCE LIFE" AND FOUND OUT THE HARD WAY THAT I WAS AN ALCOHOLIC WITH A HIGHLY ADDICTIVE PERSONALITY.

During my late teens and early twenties, I lived in a world where drugs ran my life. With no permanent residence, I lived a life that was dark with very little hope. After a period of misery and confusion, I cleaned up and got married, had a daughter, and went back to school. Believing that I was only a drug addict, I began having a glass of wine with my studies at night. This quickly escalated to drinking heavily, and I was once again falling apart—not that there was much to fall apart in the first place. A decade had passed since my "year off." Since then, I'd had three children (the first passed away, being born without kidneys). And my marriage had failed. I surrendered to the realization that I couldn't moderate or control my addictions.

So there I was, sober, divorced, with two children, with no real direction in life, and starting over. I had started working in the health and fitness industry in years prior and found a passion in helping other people get healthy and active even though I was still carrying most of the weight I had gained while on bed-rest with my first pregnancy. I started to learn to invest in myself, I lost more than 100 pounds, studied exercise science, and became a successful personal trainer.

Between teaching yoga and personal training, I absolutely loved what I was doing. I felt like I finally was able to enjoy my life. I had become active in my community and could play actively with my children until they tapped out. I had begun dating again. My life was starting to look like that of a "normal" adult.

The only drawback was that I had hit a ceiling. My days were booked up with classes and clients, and while I was making more than I ever had in my life, I knew I wanted more. I wanted to be financially stable, consistently growing my savings, putting away money for my children's future. Although I made my own schedule and had some level of flexibility, my financial obligations ultimately called the shots.

A few years ago, something devastating happened—something that changed my life. When I thought I should have been at my healthiest, my body had taken enough. I began having issues with my digestive system, I was always painfully cold, and I had no strength or energy. I was getting confused easily, and I struggled to process information. There were many other weird things happening, too. Thus began what I now call my "tour of specialists."

It took more than a dozen specialists to diagnose me. Through this journey there were just as many blessings as there were disappointments. There were times I found out more about my body than any human being should ever know, including finding a small tumor in my head, which turned out to be harmless. However, that led to a weekend of waiting, not knowing what it meant. Facing the idea of death makes you really take a long look at your life. I had some huge victories in my life. I also had things that I kept putting off until "tomorrow." Dreams like getting re-married, working for myself, impacting the world in a positive manner, and spending more time with my family. I realized that somewhere along the way I had given up on a lot of my dreams and that with my past I was lucky to just be alive and paying my bills. Wanting more from life was out of the question. Most people don't get that wake-up call.

The succession of specialists I was sent to got very tiring. I couldn't take time off of work, since of course, if I didn't work, I didn't get paid or have health insurance. I was juggling working full time, my decreasing amount of energy, and specialist appointments. There were days I would see more than one specialist, and some days I would have three or four different blood draws. The stress of not knowing, having to push through to keep my job, and endless appointments began to really take its toll.

I began trying everything I could think of to help to improve my overall health. I may not have known what was wrong, but I did know that there were areas that I could stop causing damage. I thought I lived a healthy lifestyle before I got sick, but as I started to examine it, I found many areas where I could improve. I tried different ways of eating to figure out which way made me feel the best, from vegan, to macrobiotic, to probiotic, to juicing only for almost three weeks, to eating only organic, non-processed foods. I also became aware of what I was putting on and around my body. It is crazy how many people shell out the big bucks to eat clean but douse their body in toxins and chemicals every day! I began making all of my personal care and cleaning products, which is where I really began my journey with essential oils. I had used patchouli for years as a natural perfume but had no idea how amazing essential oils really could be.

Throughout this time, I had started working from home part time for The Health Coach Group since I was unable to get out other than to go to work and appointments. Going on disability was beginning to look inevitable. I knew that I didn't want to stop working in an industry I loved, but also knew I needed to be realistic about my ability to work. Something had to change. I finally decided it was time to step back from the fitness industry, and I began working for the health coaching company full time. Being able to work from home made a big difference. It gave me the time and flexibility I needed to really take care of myself. I still found that I needed to work so many hours in order to cover my bills. At the time, I really thought this was as good as it could get.

In January 2014, I was finally diagnosed with my first diagnosis of Hyperadrenergic Postural Orthostatic Tachycardia Syndrome, a form of dysautonomia. The things in my body that were supposed to function automatically didn't always work. However, I still didn't know what was causing it.

As it happens, that was also the month that I enrolled with dōTERRA. I was still unaware of just how pure and powerful the oils were. I had gifted friends and family with some of the body products I had been making for myself over the holidays and they loved them. I wanted to share with them how they could make their own products and it seemed like the next logical step. I also started experimenting with the oils and finding the ones that would help support the systems in my body. It was amazing! I began to really play around with the oils. I wasn't creating additional stress through chemical exposure and I was really helping to support my body.

My initial goal when I signed up with my company was to get to a point where it paid for my oils each month. I didn't really consider doing it as a business and in no way did I think creating an income from it would ever be possible, especially with my limitations. I also didn't have any interest in using any of the other products—just the oils. I was comfortable there.

Then something happened. I saw how much the oils were improving my family's life in all areas: mind, body, and spirit. I really loved and trusted the company. I decided to try the supplements and found that it made a big difference in how I felt and the level of support it provided to my body. This was game-changing. As someone in the health and wellness industry, I knew it would be doing people a disservice not to educate them on how amazing these oils are. I made the decision to stop dabbling and to really do the business. Deep down, I probably knew it from the start.

On Halloween 2014, I had a surgery to repair a double hernia (common with my disorder) and didn't have to worry about not getting paid during the recovery time. It was then I realized that when I had to step away from working in a gym, I was really being given a second chance—a chance to create the flexibility and freedom that I craved in my life. I no longer had to work endlessly, wearing my body down, worrying about how many hours I needed to put in each week. I was being given the ability to really take control over my life in every aspect.

A year and a half ago, I hit a huge milestone when I made more income with dōTERRA than I had as a full-time personal trainer. I literally replaced my income while working a full-time job. I can't even tell you how amazing that is and how much pressure it alleviated. The ceiling that I hit when I was working solely in fitness? It isn't there anymore. I can continue to grow my business as large as I choose. I can be a health coach and train because I want to, without the pressure of needing to earn a certain amount to cover my bills or expenses. I don't have to worry about burnout or coaching out of necessity instead of for enjoyment and wanting to improve the lives of others. I can even nap when I need to!

In other words, I can work around my illness instead of killing myself working through it.

In early 2015, I had an amazing opportunity. I participated in a program where the company paid for my travel. I was able to travel the country teaching others about essential oils and support my team in person. I was able to visit the leaders on my team and really deepen our relationship and help them in their business. I was able to travel more in four months than I had my entire life. It was completely unreal. Words can't even describe what a life-changing experience it really was. I don't have the limitation of having to work in one place anymore. When I travel, I can bring my work with me, or I can take time for myself. The flexibility is unreal.

My quality of life has drastically improved, and I'm not only talking about the improvements to my health. I'm talking about my children each having their own bedroom in our new home, having a car that I can rely on, having time to spend with my family, being more conscious of what I am putting on and around my body and how that affects me, being able to take care of myself, being able to travel, and sharing experiences that I had given up on ever having. I am talking about really living.

When I hear about how the products have made a difference for someone else, or when I hear someone on my team ecstatically describe how they've hit a huge goal and are seeing their business flourish, the feeling is indescribable. I have formed relationships with amazing people and learned so much about life, business, resilience, and faith. I have found my path and my voice.

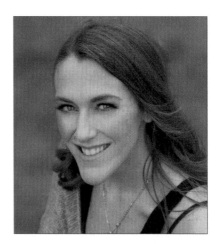

Ashlie Pappas is happily married with two children, an 8-year-old boy and a 12-year-old girl. She has been in the health and wellness industry for more than a decade as a nutrition counselor, weight loss specialist, personal trainer, yoga instructor, and health coach, and she is currently in school for aromatherapy. Ashlie has personally lost over 130 pounds. She has Ehler-Danlos Syndrome, which she manages naturally. Her personal experience with obesity and illness fuel her passion for helping others to find health, wellness, and joy in their own lives. **Learn more:** *www.ashliepappas.com; ashlie@naturallyashlie.com*

THOUGHTS ON
LEADERSHIP

by Ashlie Pappas

- Always **practice what you preach.** You can't duplicate what you aren't doing.

- **Put your leaders first.** The more you help them, the more it helps you.

- **Consistency is key.** Keep moving forward no matter what. In the big picture this can help you move mountains!

- **Self-care is a must!** If you are depleted, you have nothing to offer.

- Come from a place of **authenticity**. The heart speaks loudly.

- **Understand where others are coming from.** Help them meet *their* goals and not your goals *for* them.

- **Create systems, schedules, and stay organized.** It keeps you on track and in contact with your team.

- **Have a positive, solution-oriented mindset.** With this, you can turn seemingly bad situations into great opportunities.

- Have **FUN**!

25

FINDING REST— AND SHARING JOY

by Karina Sammons

My grandpa was a medical doctor, so pharmaceuticals were the norm when we were sick—which wasn't often. My mom was actually the first one in our family to turn into a "health nut," as we affectionately called her. She was diagnosed with a congenital heart condition, and as she researched how to care for herself, she learned the true importance of healthy food, exercise, quality supplements, and healthy living. For me, this light bulb moment eventually happened years later when I myself became a mother. Once I had precious babies counting on me, I realized I was accountable to them. My husband, Gary, and I ventured into the world of organic eating, drinking clean water, and green cleaning and started becoming increasingly conscious of what we were putting in and on our bodies.

When sweet Connor, our second child, was born at home with the assistance of my amazing hubby and two nurse-midwives, we were instantly in love with him. Our two-year-old Madelyn was so excited to have a real live baby-doll in the house! Soon after Connor was born we noticed he had a lot of digestive upset. I knew this was typical for new babies, so we just tried to roll with it. I asked many experienced mothers what they did to help their uncomfortable bundles of joy and we tried it all—just about every tip or trick that was suggested. The trouble was that although he was a happy baby, Connor had trouble sleeping comfortably.

One day in Connor's ninth month, my dear friend Betsy called. "Kari, it just occurred to me," she said. "You might want to try some of these new oils I found. There's a digestive blend that might be really helpful." By the time she finished telling me about essential oils, I was thinking, *Heck, yeah, bring on the natural plant-based stuff!* Betsy came over with a small vial of oil and coached me how to use it. That evening I rubbed one drop on Connor's tummy and put him to bed. He slept through the night!

This felt like a miracle moment for us. That next morning I stood over Connor's bed and tears dripped down my cheeks, tears of joy. In my heart I knew that we had just found something real that could significantly help our family. This was a turning point for us and the trajectory for me to learn more about essential oils and all their many uses. I felt empowered to help my family with the daily things that come about. And although Gary was skeptical for a little while, he saw my excitement and supported me trying our new oils for every little bump and scrape. And yes, eventually he learned to appreciate the many benefits the oils provided for him including boosted immunity, joint and muscle soothing, increased energy and focus, and so much more.

My famous last words to Betsy were, "I am not going to do this as a business!" But in my heart, I knew that I wouldn't be able to keep myself from sharing about these oils with the people I loved. Because she shared with me, our lives had changed overnight—literally!—and I knew so many others were looking for natural, holistic options for their own families. I felt it was my responsibility to share this good news. Something about these oils resonated deep within my heart. I knew that our Creator had given us everything we needed on this earth to keep us healthy (Ezekiel 47:12). As I dove into Bible scriptures, I was amazed how these oils were mentioned all through the text. Many were verses that I had read for much of my life but never noticed the "oils" in there! Myrrh, frankincense, sandalwood, cassia, cinnamon, cypress, and the list goes on. James 5:13-16, about anointing the sick with oil in the name of the Lord, was especially poignant to me.

These oils became a vehicle to have very real conversations that went way deeper than talking about the weather with neighbors, friends, and family. People were increasingly excited to try something all-natural for their everyday needs. And how beautiful to have these meaningful interactions and to dive into the journey together to "give it a try" with the oils, supplements, and other new products my company was releasing.

Before I knew it, we had a team, a real-live, growing, living team. And not only that, but I kept getting these checks in the mail that were more than covering the cost of our own product orders. I returned home from an essential oils convention with a new urgency to share boldly about this important health and wellness alternative. Having heard from scientists about the chemistry of the oils, I couldn't keep quiet. Gary saw my passion and supported my desire to teach regular classes and spread the love of oils one drop at a time! It would be easy to wrap up here with that cliché statement, "The rest is history."

But honestly, that's where the most important part of our story began. As much fun as I was having teaching and sharing, I knew that my biggest passion was the joy of being a mom. We also dreamed of having more time and resources to serve in our community and around the world. Gary worked hard as a corporate attorney here in Columbus, making it possible for me to be home with the kids. We didn't want my new-found passion to overshadow that, and thankfully, it didn't have to! The greatest thing about this opportunity is that you can grow it at your own pace: It's not a race. One conversation at a time (during kids' nap times), one class at a time, one follow-up phone call or appointment at a time. Our team continues to grow. And all the while, I can honestly exclaim when people ask me, "So what do you do?" my response remains, "I'm a full-time momma!" [Pause…] "And for fun, on the side, I teach health and wellness classes about how to use natural alternatives. Have you ever heard of essential oils?"

We didn't win any races to hit our ranks. Our team grew gradually. Over time, as we saw our close friends and family members who we partnered with from the very beginning grow into dynamic leaders for their own teams. Our family grew by one more too! Emily was born in April 2011 and we affectionately called her our "oil baby" because she got oiled up from the time we knew of her existence. Both our family and our organization have grown up very organically. And because of that, there's so much depth and stability as well as so many life-long relationships rooted in our love for people, natural living, and our love for Jesus, too!

"For to whom much is given, of him much shall be required. And from him to whom much was entrusted, much will be asked." Luke 12:48 was one of the verses that was read during our wedding in May 2004. Gary and I already knew at that time we had been entrusted and blessed with so much. And we were eager to give back to the people who had poured into us for our whole lives—especially, our parents—and to see some of our other dreams realized. The most dramatic dream of mine materialized in April 2014 when Gary quit his corporate law job to work side by side with me.

Wow! It was a secret dream I had kept close to my heart because I didn't know if Gary would even have that interest. But as he saw the continued, steady growth of our team, steady increases in our paychecks, and so many lives being impacted, he shared with me his desire to partner together fully in this journey. The fact that my originally very skeptical, super analytical, and uber conservative husband would confidently leave his secure job spoke volumes about the stability of our business and the larger company.

It's been well over two years now, and we joyfully exclaim it's been the best decision! Our kids always have one of us "on" with them, and then we flip-flop job shifts. We've had fun finding our new normal, and our kids have flourished having daddy around more often. I have, too!

And as our children and our business continue to mature, we are finding more opportunities to give and serve as a family. It seems like everywhere we turn, so many people are eager to have these beautiful oils, but so many don't have the financial resources. What a joy to give away what we have been so abundantly blessed with. We have an extremely generous team who is always eager to donate and serve where oils are needed. Currently our team is partnering with GiveOils.org and sending donations all over the globe. Additionally we look forward to the day when our kids can join us on the Healing Hands Foundation trips. Meanwhile, we are in the process of dreaming up and organizing several local and international service projects for our team.

It has been an amazing privilege during these past months adding new visions, goals, and partnerships to our list—and to see them already being realized. Having our three kids with us on a recent company incentive trip, along with my parents, Mark and Lori Vaas, and so many close friends, felt like a full-circle moment, especially as we were all digging in the dirt together planting ginger. The fact that this "job" is creating so many opportunities not only for our family but for people around the globe, while growing real health and financial freedom is priceless.

That God planted this opportunity right in our lap has been a great honor. I am so glad we didn't dismiss it. Our greatest joy is seeing lives changed every day because someone shared the love of oils. It's that simple. Just open up the bottle, breathe in, and savor it. And then share the blessing with someone you love. You won't regret it.

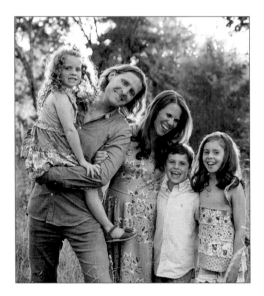

Karina Sammons and her husband Gary have been married for 12 years and live in Ohio. Karina has never felt like an oils "sales person"; she has simply created a new way to share her love for those around her. Between the Sammons' faith, sharing essential oils with others, and raising their three children, Karina is living a life she loves. **Learn more: www.team healthyessentials.com.**

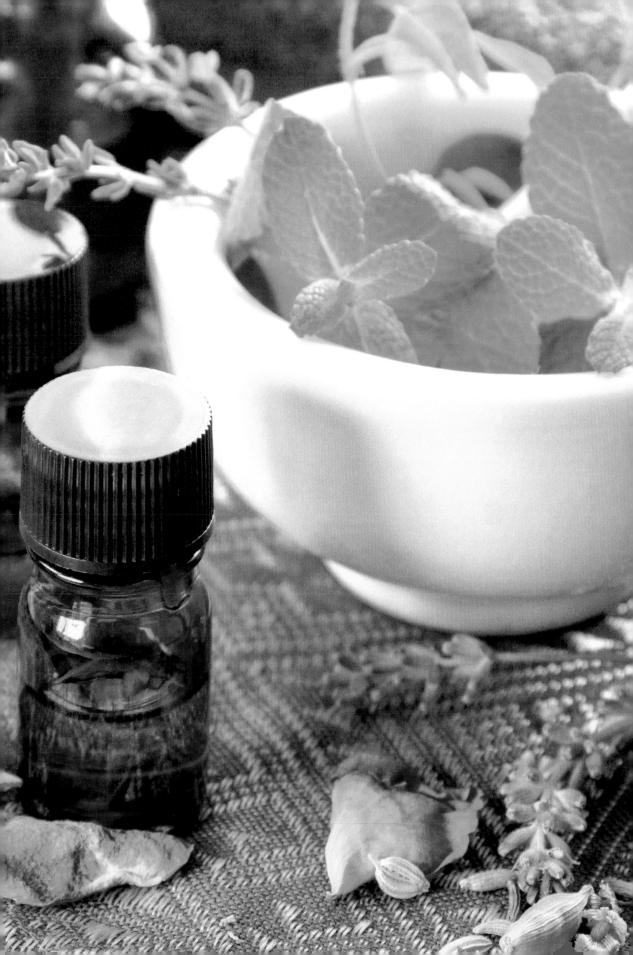

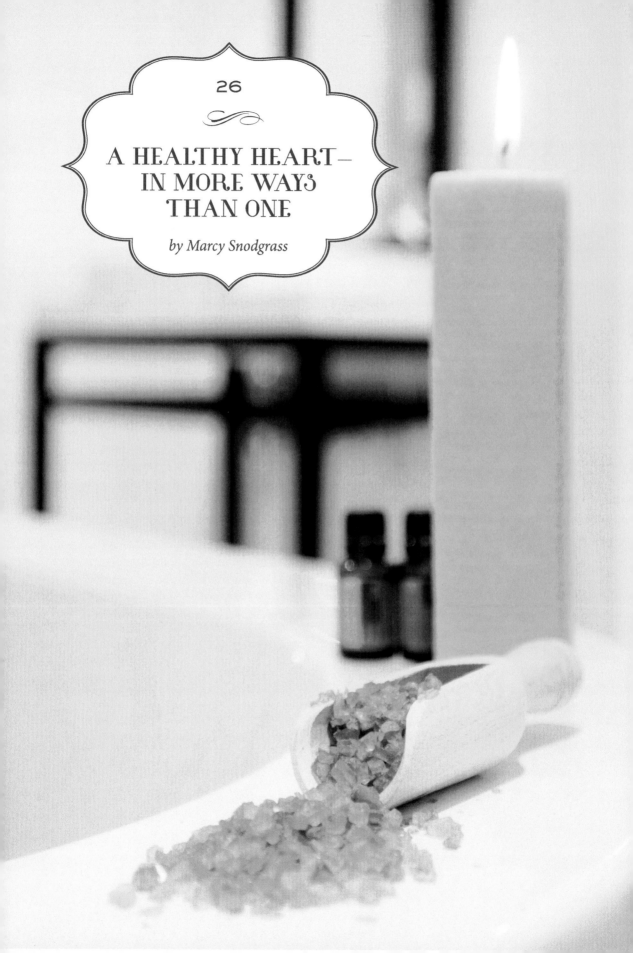

26

A HEALTHY HEART—
IN MORE WAYS
THAN ONE

by Marcy Snodgrass

I share my story so that you may know that there is a way out of misery. If you are experiencing this, know that you are not alone.

"You need open heart surgery again."

These were the words that rang in my ears. I had my first open heart surgery at the age of twenty-three, when I received an artificial carotid artery due to inflammation of the arteries. I had been on steroids and immune suppressants for several years already, and I had been diagnosed with osteopenia, the beginnings of brittle bones, because of the medications.

Doctors told me this would be the rest of my life. I was thirty pounds overweight, and it was all I could do to get out of bed and go to work every day. I had no energy, was in pain all day, and felt the turmoil inside constantly. I felt mentally stressed most days. All those things were side effects of the medications, and of my disease, Takayasu's arteritis.

I owned and operated a spa and salon that was on Salon Today's Top 200 fastest growing list for five years, so it appeared I had everything running smoothly to the outside world. But on the inside, I was falling apart. Those closest to me—my family—knew I struggled. But, even they didn't know the full extent of my physical and mental pain.

From the very beginning, I was supposed to have been stillborn or have had severe brain damage. But I was born healthy and whole. When I was two years old, my parents discovered that I had an egg allergy, because I nearly died from a severe reaction to one bite of scrambled egg. Then, I had heart surgery in my early twenties.

Ongoing medical procedures, along with some youthful spending decisions, had left my husband and I in a world of financial debt. I was sick, miserable, and broke. I felt broken.

However, when I heard those words from the doctor, there was this seed of hope in me, because of my faith in God. I knew God loved me and that my life had purpose.

I knew there had to be a better way, and I couldn't stand the thought of going through another surgery. I asked the doctors to give me six months to work on it myself. They reluctantly said yes, and in return, I agreed to be checked regularly to make sure it wasn't getting any worse. As a massage therapist, I was open to holistic and alternative medicine, so I decided to go that route.

I had three goals:
1. Practice yoga
2. Change my nutrition
3. Receive more body work

Over time, my body, my mind, and my spirit started to change in positive ways. I lost the weight, I had more energy, I began to feel back to myself again, and my bone scan returned to normal after a year and a half of working this plan. They began to reduce my medications very slowly.

I transitioned my way nutritionally as well. I began by eating less burgers and pizza and more healthy food, organic food and, finally, juicing. I continued to receive more body therapies.

My husband and I took a financial planning course, and with really hard work, brought ourselves out of debt. These new habits became a way of life. Over time, I became a yoga instructor, a holistic health coach, and an organic juice bar owner. But this didn't happen overnight. It took years.

I believe we are so conditioned to think everything has a quick fix, so we forget that it takes time and dedication to change our minds and bodies. If we really put the effort in, we will see change.

It took about seven years, but I finally came off of all of the medications the doctors said I would be on forever. I will never forget the day the doctor called to tell me I could come off of the last dose of steroid they had kept me on for so long. It had been such a long road. My youngest son was about fourteen at the time, and when I hung up the phone, the emotions overwhelmed me, and I burst into tears. My son asked me what was wrong, and I said, "These are tears of joy, baby. Tears of a long hard journey." It seems impossible to even describe the emotion that ran through me. I had changed my life through God's strength!

Through my journey, I have realized that every single person has the ability to have a huge impact on their own health. It's not magic, and it doesn't happen overnight, but you can absolutely change your life.

Our bodies have such an amazing ability when we treat them right and put healthy things in and on our bodies and in our minds. Attitude is so important.

I love that quote by Henry Ford: "If you think you can, or you think you can't, you're right."

As I took my health into my own hands, it became clear to me what my mission needed to be. I was here to help others see that they, too, have an amazing ability to improve their lives, both physically and financially. I wanted a way to empower others that felt authentic to me.

We all have opportunities to create financial health. But for some reason, money continues to be a big issue for many people. I find this so disheartening. And, this is where my dōTERRA story begins...

Why do we not feel worthy to have money?

And it goes deeper.

Why do we not feel worthy to live the life we desire?

The truth is, there is nothing wrong with money, or having financial security and abundance. We have been conditioned by our culture and our circumstances to live in a scarcity mindset. But think of it this way: The more money we make, the more we can give. Think of all the good we can do in the world when we have a proper relationship with money.

My mission is to help other women become physically and financially abundant. I am a certified health coach, and as I train people on ways to use nutrition to feel good, I also found a great essential oil company to expand my business. I have shared essential oils with people as a massage therapist for years, but it has become more of the focus in my work over the last couple of years. It is such a gift to be able to share something as amazing as essential oils and focus a career around something I love so much. It's so fun! I love witnessing people have an a-ha moment the first time they have an experience with essential oils. It's a certain smile, and I know they've got it.

Every time I teach a workshop on essential oils, I am amazed that there are new people attending who are thirsty for knowledge. I could work 24x7 answering questions, or, I can give people the resources they need to find the answers. I choose the latter. I love empowering people in that way! It allows me to live a life I love. I have the freedom to spend time with my family, go on vacation at the spur of a moment, make my own schedule, and hang out with very good friends—my team members. What more could I ask for?

What I love the most is that dōTERRA has allowed me to really step into a leadership role. As a leader, I teach others how to build a team, and how to get out of debt, feel supported, and live a resourced life.

I have learned that we each have the power to make our lives look the way we want it to look. We can work ourselves to death, or we can work strategically and really create a life we love. I have learned that I have the choice to allow my business to be "big enough" when I need it to be, or to push for the next level, without sacrificing my family and relationships.

My, how my life has changed over the years! I love being present in each moment, and I look forward to the next step in my business and adventures. My oldest son is in the military, and my youngest is a senior in high school. Looks like my husband and I have some fun years ahead, and there is no doubt in my mind that dōTERRA is a big part of that and a great tool to fuel my passion for people.

Marcy Snodgrass is a vibrant, fun health coach, yoga instructor, and entrepreneur who loves life! She loves teaching people how to live their best life, with physical and financial freedom. Marcy has 25 years of experience using essential oils, and shares that knowledge in a light-hearted, easy way. Her positive attitude is infectious. Being in a class with Marcy will leave you feeling grounded, inspired, and ready to create a life you love! **Learn more: www.marcysnodgrass.com; msnodgrass@ hotmail.com.**

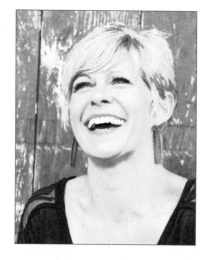

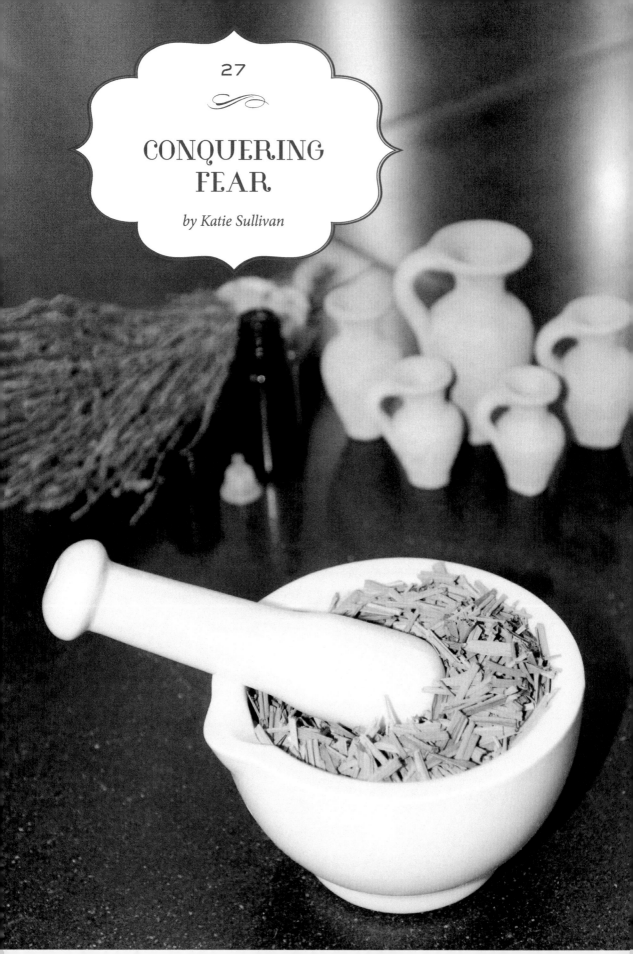

27

CONQUERING FEAR

by Katie Sullivan

MY STORY OF FINDING TRUE HEALTH AND EMPOWERMENT BEGAN ON A PADDLEBOARD IN THE PACIFIC OCEAN OFF MAUI; WAS ALMOST DERAILED EIGHTY-NINE FEET BELOW THE OCEAN'S SURFACE IN MEXICO; TOOK AN UNEXPECTED PIT STOP IN LYON, FRANCE; AND FINALLY CAME TO FULL FRUITION ON MY URBAN FARM IN ARIZONA, WHERE I WAS ABLE TO FINALLY PUT ALL THE PIECES TOGETHER. LET ME EXPLAIN.

I have been active my whole life. I have five beautiful children, and in 2012 I enrolled in a yoga teacher training program, which I completed the following year. Health-wise I was in great shape. But personally I was still feeling defeated, tired, and powerless. Shortly after graduating from the yoga teacher training program, I took a trip to Hawaii. I have always been scared of water and, up to that point, wouldn't even swim in my pool with my kids. But on a particular sunny morning in Maui in 2013 I found myself on a paddleboard in the middle of the Pacific Ocean and was asked, dared, whatever, as the yoga teacher in the group, to do a headstand on it. I had never done one away from the safety of a wall or where I hadn't fallen completely over away from a wall—let alone on a rocking paddleboard in the middle of a body of water that terrified me—but I decided I would go for it. The next five minutes set my life on a new path. I rocked that headstand. What I felt was impossible had just become possible. I had just done it.

I came home from that trip still terrified of water, and so I decided to do what all people terrified of water do—sign up for a PADI open water scuba diving class. It would be an understatement to say it was the hardest thing I had ever done. If my anxiety had been an airport, it would have been Code Orange. I persevered and completed the classwork and pool dives and found myself headed back to Maui a month later to complete my certification—and I did! The impossible had become the possible, again. I had done it.

One year later, I decided to go for my PADI advanced open water scuba diving certification. I was still afraid of water, but this time I was open-water diver certified with a handful of dives logged. I was in Mexico, and my first dive went fine.

The second dive is where everything came undone. Seventy feet below the surface during a routine dive to complete the necessary deep dive for advanced certification, my instructor, his dive buddy, myself, and my dive buddy became trapped in a down current. In seconds we were pulled to eighty-nine feet below surface level. It was like being trapped in the world's largest washing machine; the current was so strong our air bubbles pulled downward.

For me, it was every fear come to fruition. Five beautiful children at home, so many things I wanted to do with them that were away from my computer that had not been done, so many regrets from the past few years while I had been trying to navigate my forties and what I wanted. Is *this* where it would end for me? In the Sea of Cortez eighty-nine feet below the surface? Luckily for me, I was with a Master diver who was able to get us to the surface. Lucky for me, I had completed a yoga teacher training course and had breathing and mind-calming techniques to keep me from completely panicking while he worked to save us. These factors saved my life that day. It was not lost on me how close we four divers had come to being the next day's lead news story. My instructor said later he ran it back through his mind several times—each time, coming up with a scenario that ended with dead bodies.

My instructor, in his wisdom, decided I needed to get back in the water the next day or forever be stuck in all my previous fears of water, all now completely compounded in the knowledge of having nearly drowned the day before. John Wayne was quoted as saying "Courage is being scared to death… and saddling up anyway." It was time to saddle up. On the boat ride to the diving spot, I had an epiphany: If I wanted my life to be different, then from this day forward I was going to have to take proactive steps to live the life I truly wanted.

I had another realization that day. I had spent my whole life up to that point living in fear of one kind or another, typically centered on thoughts of not being good enough. I knew this wasn't what God wanted for me. He didn't want me to have fear—not above or below the water. It was time to trust God's plan for my life, and it was time to take a proactive role in creating the life I truly wanted.

The next ten hours would find me completing three boat dives and one shore dive that included my longest timed dive to date and a night dive. The impossible had just become the impossible again. I came home from that trip, completed one more necessary dive, and the woman who wouldn't swim in her pool fourteen months earlier had officially become a certified PADI advanced open water scuba diver.

The reaction to a near-death experience, I'm assuming, is different for everyone. For me, it encouraged me in some areas and forced me to make changes in others. Specifically, even though I had a successful nineteen-year career as a speech-language pathologist, that was no longer my bliss; it was time to take a much needed break. Besides my family, what I truly loved was holistic health, writing, and traveling. It was time to put my energy into something that I was passionate about and release those endeavors that were no longer adding to my happiness, no matter how good at them I was. I initially revamped my travel blog and thought about how I could add holistic health into its mission. As a registered yoga teacher and a certified level 2 Reiki practitioner I had a good start. The final piece came when I rekindled my love for natural healthcare.

In September 2014, I had a day that started at an appointment with a traditional Chinese herbalist and ended at a large natural market. I came home and realized it had been a joy-filled day. Holistic health was my bliss. I started seeking other ways to add holistic health into my daily life. By coincidence, I was introduced to essential oils at that same time and purchased an enrollment kit from dōTERRA. While I had first started using essential oils (from the fancy grocery store) in 2010 to make my own cleaners, I didn't know a lot about them. My enrollment came with multiple resources including how they might be incorporated into an income. I found myself using them daily, and while my transition to a natural lifestyle continued to progress, my journey to live my authentic truth was still stalling.

The following month, on the second day of a four-country, sixteen-day European road trip with my family, we pulled into Lyon, France. By 11 a.m., I was in the emergency room... in a foreign country. Lying in a hospital in a foreign country, with a large language barrier, and feeling sicker than I ever had in my life was another wake-up call. Life is precious! I needed to quit thinking about the changes I wanted to make in my life and start proactively making them. My condition improved, the trip continued, and I spent the rest of the trip doing some much needed soul searching.

Back home in Arizona, I found myself making changes, step by step. I took some time to think about my life goals at this stage in my life and what I really wanted for myself and my family. I wanted—no, I *needed*—an endeavor, a life, I could be excited about again. It took a little time to figure out what direction I wanted to go, but it was worth it to make sure I was moving in the right direction for my long-term happiness. In 2015, I had my answer and a new endeavor I was completely passionate about. I tied my experience and credentials for travel, holistic health, yoga, and natural living together and started a travel and yoga lifestyle blog called rebelplum.

Today, water doesn't scare me anymore. My love for natural living has grown to include making my own spa and beauty products with essential oils and working on an herbalist certification. After a much needed break, I still see clients as a Speech-Language Pathologist, but now I feel passion, not burnout. I love it all. I'm living my truth.

I think back to that day on the paddleboard. Scared. Unhappy. The feeling of powerlessness to change my life path in my forties. It seemed impossible. But it wasn't. I'm the proof it is possible. I did it.

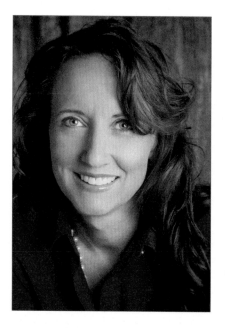

*Katie Sullivan, M.S., SLP-CCC, RYT-200, is an avid traveler, a Speech-Language Pathologist, a licensed yoga teacher, a Reiki level 2 practitioner, and a certified PADI advanced open-water scuba diver. Katie pens the travel and yoga lifestyle blog rebelplum (**www.rebelplum.com**) and provides holistic health services including sharing her love of essential oils via her business. Katie resides with her family in the beautiful Southwest, where she is currently turning her one-acre property into a European-inspired urban farm based on her travels. She writes about intentional parenting at **www.mysweethomeschool.com** and has been featured in Hobby Farm Home and Lucky magazines. **Learn more: www.rebelplum.com; rebelplum77@gmail.com.***

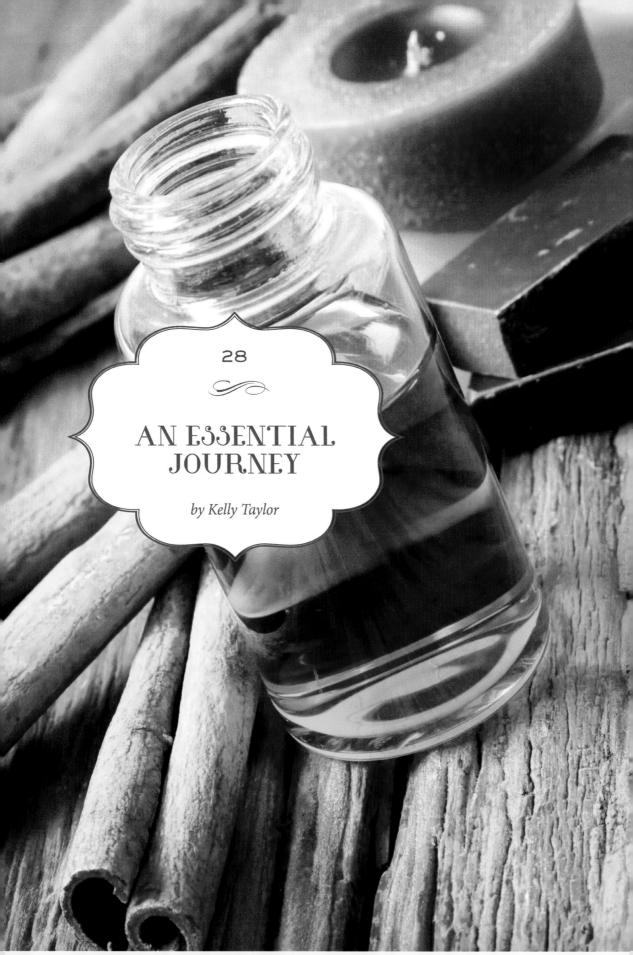

28

AN ESSENTIAL
JOURNEY

by Kelly Taylor

Today I get goosebumps when a friend or client calls to thank me for helping them learn to live healthier lives. Because, for more than 20 years, my husband and I owned and operated an ice cream restaurant, specializing in burgers, fries, and ice cream cakes. This didn't exactly facilitate healthy eating. By 2008, with two kids onboard, we realized that as a family we needed to get serious about our health, so my handsome husband and I committed to a better diet and added as much exercise into our days as possible. He lost close to 100 pounds, and I lost more than 40 pounds.

However, losing weight isn't half as hard as keeping it off. If we were really committed to living better lives—and we were—we needed to live a life without daily temptation of homemade ice cream, warm brownies, and steak sandwiches! And we wanted more meaningful time with our kids, too. And so, we sold the business. Not long after, I enrolled at the Institute for Integrative Nutrition and became a certified Health Coach, which only fueled and supported my passion for a healthier lifestyle—not just for myself and my family but for all those around me. I continued to educate myself in all things healthy and became certified in Plant-Based Nutrition and as a Raw Food Chef and Instructor.

Through all this, my life was consumed with an even bigger health issue—and the emotional repercussions.

Back when we still had the ice-cream restaurant, our youngest son suddenly began losing his sight. I can't even describe the terror my husband and I felt when we realized the extent of issues our son was facing. It was beyond our comprehension! We couldn't have been more devastated to learn of the complete diagnoses: a very rare brain disease called Batten's Disease that causes blindness early on and the effects continue to evolve without hope for a cure.

Never before had I seen my life flash before me, yet out of all the chaos came a new level of determination. How could this be true? He was a very bright, active kid. We weren't going to take the doctor's word as the path for his future. Instead, we decided to find ways to better manage his symptoms. We were going to beat the odds, or at least live every minute completely balls-out awesome!

While I focused on helping our son have all of the opportunities, experiences, and the best life he could while balancing family needs, I had an innate drive to seek accomplishment and was always dreaming of ways to learn new useful things. And one of those new things was essential oils. That, it turns out, was the missing link in my life.

We live in a very small town so I knew it would benefit me to create an online business that I could access and take anywhere. I'd had success with the ice cream shop in my tiny town of 500, but obviously essential oils were a whole different ballgame.

I have learned that people need support and solutions for real issues. They need an advocate who cares and who will take the time to listen—and that's me! I love listening to people and helping them in ways I never dreamed possible. I have always been a problem solver, coming up with ways to work things out with everyone's best interest taken into consideration. I love helping people realize they have the power within them to take control of a situation in their lives that seems out of touch, whether that is their health, happiness, or finances. What I am doing now, completely on my terms, is awesome.

And it all started with deciding to sell a business that was making money. It was one of the most difficult decisions I've ever made, even though it took up so much of my time. You know what running an ice-cream business means? No summers!

My happiest places to be are poolside on a hot summer day or on a Caribbean beach with my family swimming with sea turtles! I could have hired a manager and let them run the business, but then I wouldn't have been making the kind of money I wanted for all the responsibility that was still inevitably mine.

Selling the business taught me it is okay to be scared of not knowing what will come next, but if you don't make a change you will never know what you could be missing out on. Life is meant to be lived, not looked back upon. I am thankful every day for choosing to take the leap into very uncertain waters with my husband by my side encouraging me all the way.

Now I travel and share essential oils with new friends all over the country. I enjoy every minute of this amazing and precious life! I love what I do, and when I share from my heart, I experience a bigger version of success than I could ever have imagined.

I get to communicate daily with people on my team and with new friends that I meet online or in local classes. I also get to help my team reach financial freedom and meet their own goals by supporting them to build their essential oils businesses. All around, essential oils have blessed my family and myself, and I could not be more thankful.

With my home-based business, many days go by when I don't even leave my beautiful home, but the awesome part is that I don't *have* to. I have everything I need right here!

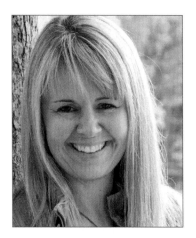

*Kelly Taylor is a Diamond Wellness Advocate with dōTERRA International and has enjoyed sharing dōTERRA essential oils with her family and friends for over four years. Kelly attended school at the Institute of Integrated Nutrition and became a certified Health Coach in 2010. She is also certified in the AromaTouch™ Technique, is a T. Colin Campbell Plant-Based Nutrition graduate, and a member of the American Association of Drugless Practitioners. Starting her own business with dōTERRA, Kelly was offered the freedom that was miss-ing in her previous business endeavors. Kelly now enjoys working hard and spending time with her two sons and loving husband at their beautiful home in Penn-sylvania. **Learn more:** www.kellytaylorwellness.com; hello@kellytaylorwellness.com*

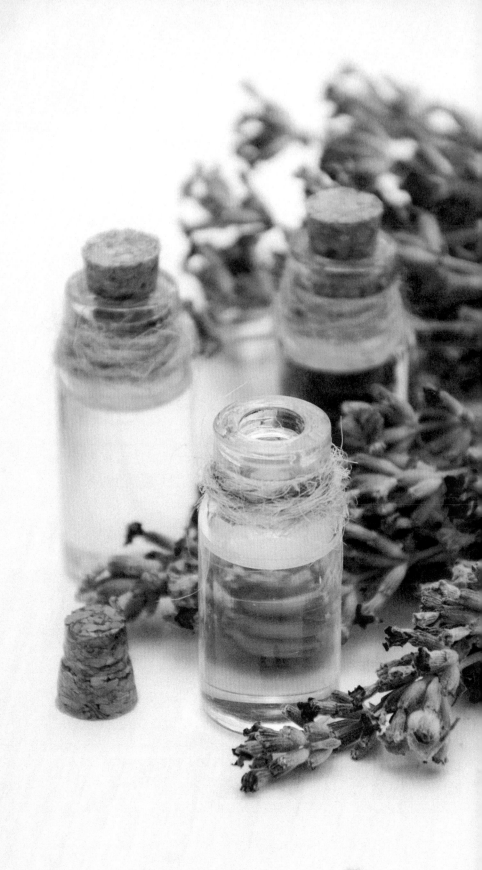

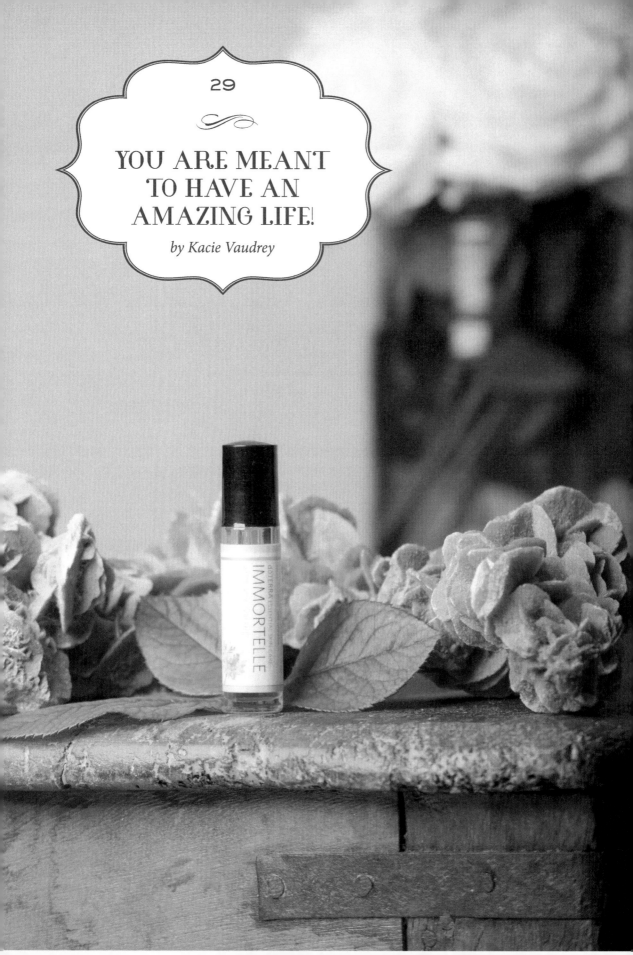

29

YOU ARE MEANT TO HAVE AN AMAZING LIFE!

by Kacie Vaudrey

My story is about a simple girl who learned to live through chaos, seek love, and find peace in abundance. It's funny how life works, and I have needed to laugh many times on my crazy ride! We are all given the exact same tools and opportunity to lead an amazing life. Great, there's hope for all of us. We plan. We seek. We dream. And just about the time we *think* we have it all figured out we are thrown a curve ball that leads us down a path we never imagined as our destiny. Curve balls, generally speaking, don't have a place in our plan. Or do they? Are they the missing link that forces us out of our comfort zone and into a place of abundance and growth, leading us to the greater good of our existence?

Here's the thing. Curve balls come in many forms. The good. The bad. The UGLY. Two years ago I was faced with illness and divorce. I remember thinking to myself, "Really? I'm thirty-eight years old and on a mission to help the world. Couldn't you wait a year or two?"

Silly question, really, because curve balls have no emotional connection to me or what I am currently going through. They do, however, have intention. It forced me to stop living on autopilot and missing the things in life that matter. I was pushed to be a better person, better business partner, to love unconditionally, and to see the good in everyone around me. I learned to smile more, laugh louder, soak up the sun, give more hugs, and love the life I was given.

"Courage is being scared to death, but saddling up anyway."

—John Wayne

Curve balls leave us deflated. Exhausted. Ready to throw in the towel. I felt that way for a split second or two… until I realized I had too much to do to give up now. I had two little kids relying on me, a business that I wasn't done building, and a love story I deserved to experience. I had options, a lot of them really. I just had to search my heart, embrace the gifts that were given to me, and keep reminding myself that something that really *stinks* could actually be an opportunity…

You see, life leaves clues for those who are awake enough to listen. It's a little something like jumping into a freezing lake. We can slowly dip our toe in to test the water or we can dive in and embrace the experience at hand. *We* get to choose. And it's when we make the choice to *not* allow challenges to dictate how our story goes that the true magic begins. We are all given the same tools to lead an amazing life; sometimes we just have to adjust, refocus, and get back to our dream to realize the true power that lives within.

Two years ago I made a choice. I opted to live. I allowed myself to awaken to the possibilities that exist within. In that moment when I allowed my suffering to subside, I realized that the past couple of years have brought growth, strength, beauty, and love to my life, and so I made a decision: Today, I file my curve balls away in their own special spot. They no longer have a place in my heart. Today they have found a new home, not because I want to forget them but more because I don't need them anymore. They have taught me everything I need to know about life and business, and now, I move forward.

Today I spend my time CELEBRATING. GROWING. LOVING. AND HELPING THE WORLD.

What do I do now?

My choice came down to saddling up or giving up. And because of the necessity of this choice, I have been able to make a massive shift in my personal life as well as in my essential oil business. I have come to realize there is no need to overcomplicate things and dwell on the past. We can find peace in the gifts that are given to us—and there are no bad ones. Detours are part of living. We build meaningful relationships, honor ourselves, and dream of a better future. We begin to live the life we are meant to live!

My journey has led me to six foundational pieces that I inherently incorporate into my daily life and into my business. I am honored to share them in hopes they will help you, too.

1. **Live with intention.** Everything we do must have a purpose. Everyone is too busy being a mother, wife, carpooler, cook, housekeeper, counselor, mentor, leader, and business-woman to live any other way. Choose your daily actions, the people you spend your time with, the activities you complete in your business, the places you go, and the things you say, and do so wisely. Make every action count, and you will create the reality you envision.

2. **Be present.** The only way we can find joy in our surroundings is by being present and enjoying the moment. Turn technology off. Stop thinking about other places or things. Share some love. Take the time to hand-write a card to celebrate a successful month, or make a phone call to offer encouragement to someone who needs a loving touch. Engage in a conversation, and listen to every word being spoken. It's easy to overlook all of the wonderful things that are happening around us when we get caught up in our own thoughts. Make the choice to never miss another beat.

3. **Build relationships.** We meet many people in our lives, and if you want to be a Presidential Diamond–level networker, you will take every opportunity to connect. Some acquaintances become life-long friends and others pass through our lives on a daily basis. There is no way to know what an individual will bring to the table. Take a risk. Don't judge. Ask a lot of questions, and enjoy the abundance that comes from building strong healthy relationships with the people you meet.

4. **Lead with your heart.** Our jobs, ultimately, revolve around love—not numbers or goals or checkmarks in a column. Love means we seek to help individuals with their current physical, emotional, spiritual, and financial health, and so many are relying on us to be their solution. We must approach our business and lives with integrity, honesty, kindness, loyalty, love, and an open heart. We must be conscious of what we are saying, how we are building, and who we are recruiting to join us on our mission. Be the example.

5. **Celebrate!** Life isn't always predictable. We all are on the same twisty road, and the curves are slippery. We think we have everything under control but then we slip off. We have all been there, and it's what we take from the experience that molds us into the

powerful individuals we become. That's the beauty of life. We are all survivors in this world together, courageous and powerful. Celebrate every single person in your life for who they are, the beauty in their heart, and their essential connection to you. Don't wait until later. Start the cheers right now!

6. Hold tight to your peaceful heart... At the end of the day we must maintain peace in our hearts. We must know that all of our daily activities and conversations were impactful and honest. Every word we say must settle in our souls. The power is in us. We have the strength to impact the world.

> *"Your work is meant to be exciting, and you are meant to accomplish all the things you would love to accomplish. Your relationships with your family and friends are meant to be filled with happiness. You are meant to have all the money you need to live a full, wonderful life. You are meant to be living your dreams—all of them!"*
>
> —Rhonda Byrne

If I could count all the ways life hasn't worked in my favor I'd be here all day. The reality is this: Life isn't pretty. If it were, things would be stagnant. Boring. There wouldn't be growth or change. There simply wouldn't be hope. Embrace every single moment and begin to live your life in new way—and remember we are all given the same tools to lead an amazing life.

Kacie Vaudrey's trail started in the west. She grew up in Wyoming, taught English for eight years at Montana State, and created two fabulous kids— Emma and Sulli. Essential oils and the benefits that they offer are part of Kacie's lifestyle, and her passion for living set fire to her business, Peaceful Heart Leadership. Kacie is a Presidential Diamond in dōTERRA with over 30,000 wellness advocates in her organization.As a trailblazer, Kacie's path is fun, fulfilling and rich with the scent of life's essence... Her secret? Finding your own Peaceful Heart and leading from that place. Learn more: www.PeacefulHeartLeadership.com; kacie@ PeacefulHeartLeadership.com.

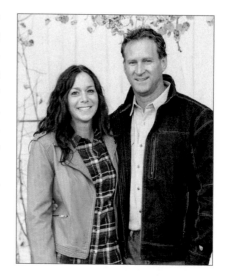

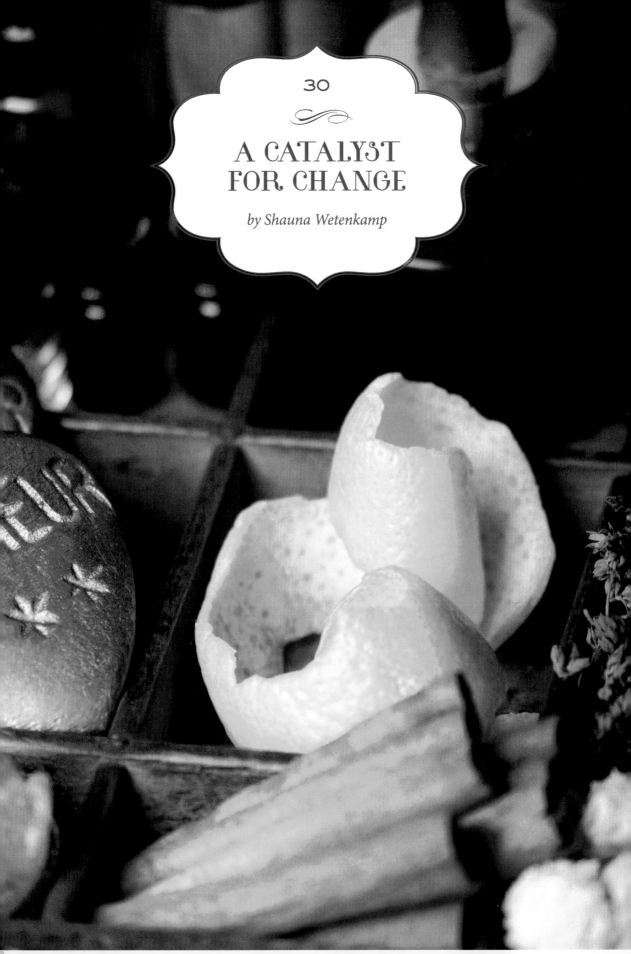

30

A CATALYST FOR CHANGE

by Shauna Wetenkamp

I decided to choose my essential oil company *for* the business opportunity. In fact, I made that decision before I had even tried a single oil. To my surprise, what was hiding inside the business opportunity wasn't the check, the oils, or even the people. It was the possibility to take myself to a place I never imagined existed.

I love my life! I have four amazing kids and a freakin' awesome hubby, and they have been my number-one fans and biggest teachers. Life puts experiences, people, and things in your path for a reason. Thankfully, I finally listened. Here's a small window into me.

I've been selling essential oils since September 2011. Looking back at all that I have experienced, it feels like it has been much longer. I have truly seen the power of these oils and, more importantly to me, I saw the power of myself. It was a catalyst for me to be what I wanted to be.

My Auntie Lona had been talking about these oils for a few months and was trying to tell me how awesome they are and how good the business opportunity was. I didn't pay much attention because she had been involved in other network marketing companies and I just thought it would be the same. To her credit, she knew our financial need and saw the potential of not just the company but the potential in me. I can see that now, although I didn't so much see it then. So I begrudgingly told my husband about Auntie Lona's new venture.

I remember exactly where I was standing, at the bottom of the stairs, when he said, "Shauna, maybe you should look into it, because if you found something you're passionate about, I know you would be really good at it." That was enough for me. I felt a flood of joy come over me when he said that, and to this day it sticks with me. He has always seen my goodness and potential, and his encouraging words meant so much to me.

We ordered a kit full of oils. When it first arrived, I saw all those oils and I never thought I would ever use them all, especially Frankincense! Who uses that?

I used the whole kit up in three weeks.

I jumped right in full speed ahead with the business and taught classes, gave out samples, followed up, and repeated the whole process. I also spoke very confidently about everything that my company had to offer and was fearless when talking to people about joining me in this business. My desire for financial success drove me to really push! I was very consistent and focused on my goal.

Two months into my journey, things started to shift when I realized the true power of these oils. I saw family members have more balanced emotions, and I saw myself giving and serving in a way that was bringing a softness to me. One of these moments was when I sat down and rubbed my mom's sore feet with Deep Blue, Frankincense, and Balance. The oils allowed me the opportunity for service and allowed me to strengthen my relationship with my mom. If I never made a dime with this business, it would be okay, because it changed my relationship with her! I then started sharing with even more passion and feeling.

A few more months went by. I had built my business and had very quickly noticed that there were naysayers all around, both in life and in business. I struggled to not take it personally, and I really started to question why I had decided to do this business. I hit a wall and let negativity get me down. My business wasn't growing, and I wasn't growing. I needed to decide if I was going to keep doing it or let others win. I was so discouraged, and the old familiar self-doubt was creeping in. I hit one of the lowest points in my life. Although I had made progress and great strides with my business, I still had to learn how to be safe and happy in this world.

I took a good long look in the mirror, and I didn't love the person looking back at me. In fact, I didn't even *know* the person who was looking back at me. I decided to turn back to things that I had started learning years earlier, and I furthered my education and personal development. I am constantly in awe of the opportunities dōTERRA provides. I have seen lives literally transformed, beginning with my own life. For me, it had really become a journey of personal development, and my "why" had become even clearer. Understanding why you are making a choice can drive you during these times! Now, when I get down, I use a mantra:

When things get hard, it drives you and guides you.

I realized my "why" was me! I had to believe in myself, care about myself, and challenge myself—and this business was helping me to change. In that moment, I made a huge shift in my life and put myself on the top of my list. I let go of friendships and relationships that were no longer serving me. I set aside time to spend with my husband and family. And I set up boundaries that I didn't even know existed before. I began to live by a great quote from Chinese philosopher and poet, Lao Tzu: "He who knows others is wise. He who knows himself is enlightened."

Once I truly started down this path, I hit the rank of Diamond. It is no longer a surprise to me to see that as you grow, your business grows! As you serve, things just fall into place. And as you find yourself, others turn to you and see and feel that strength while they're finding themselves.

I now get the chance to teach others not only about oils but about life, balance, and who they are. Using oils for physical, mental, emotional, and spiritual growth speeds up the healing process! It happened for myself and I've seen it happen for so many others. Here are some of the things that helped me on my path.

Oil Combinations I Love:
- Ylang Ylang and Geranium: in a yummy bath with a good book
- Ginger, Lime, and Bergamot: diffuse to help you get out of bed
- Frankincense and Peppermint: meditate with this delicious combo
- TerraShield® and Arborvitae: block negativity—and bugs! (wear, diffuse, spray all around)
- Immortelle and Melissa: helps raise your vibration (on heart)

Books You Just Have to Read:
- *The Alchemist,* Paulo Coelho (metaphysical fiction)
- *The Power of Receiving: A Revolutionary Approach to Giving Yourself the Life You Want and Deserve,* Amanda Owen
- *The Big Leap: Conquer Your Fear and Take Life to the Next Level,* Gay Hendricks, Ph.D.
- *The Law of Divine Compensation: On Work, Money, and Miracles,* Marianne Williamson
- *The Game of Life and How to Play It,* Florence Scovel Shinn
- *Go Pro: 7 Steps to Becoming a Network Marketing Professional,* Eric Worre

Things You Just Have to Try or Do:
- Read, pray, meditate, journal, practice yoga, foot zone therapy, reiki, EFT, chakra balancing, crystals

More Recommendations:
- Get a morning routine!
- Say no to people (No is a complete sentence!)
- Go for walks.
- Put screens—phone, computer, TV—away for good chunks of time.
- Eat lunch by yourself. Be your own best friend.
- Make time for a weekly date with your spouse or partner.
- Learn to block your energy.

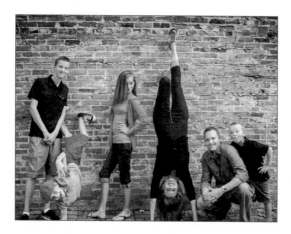

*Shauna Wetenkamp is a certified Holistic Health Coach, Emotional Facilitator, and lifetime student of the human race. She is a Blue Diamond–ranked product consultant for dōTERRA and has a passion for learning and teaching natural remedies, with a special emphasis on the emotional benefits of essential oils. She teaches classes and seminars on this subject throughout the United States. Her practice is focused on oils and other modalities including meditation, fitness, counseling, and helping people to become their best selves. Shauna lives in Central Valley California with her husband and four children. **Learn more:** www.soulfuldelights.net; loveeeedoterra@gmail.com.*

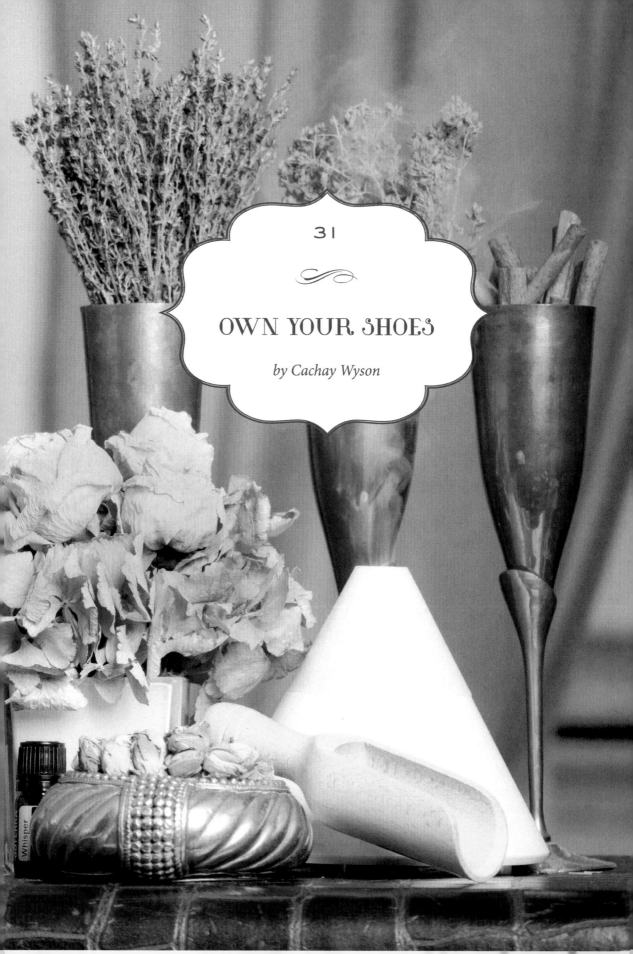

31

OWN YOUR SHOES

by Cachay Wyson

The next morning, in my exhaustion, I tried essential oils—and was empowered by the results. After that, I felt like a scientist doing experiment after experiment to see if the oils really could do this or that. My husband Joey even showed a bit of interest as he flipped through the book I was reading and saw there were things to "wake me up and get me in the mood." After giggling about that far-off hope from this recovering momma, he seemed to not be so resistant to the idea of using essential oils.

With my main business degree being in Homemaking, with a minor in Motherhood, self taught, I was not looking for a business opportunity. The dōTERRA opportunity found me anyway, and I had a choice to either step out into a place that was uncomfortable and share or keep this gem to myself staying in my comfort zone.

Our family became empowered with dōTERRA essential oils, and people around us were noticing, asking questions, and looking for further information. I set a goal to get my oils paying for themselves, because I didn't believe it was in our budget to continue purchasing essential oils monthly. Having a false belief that I "couldn't sell," I would share but shy away from how they could get their own wholesale account. But then, switching my beliefs from "I can't sell" to "I can educate" empowered me to start sharing with people and get them their own wholesale account one by one. I believed I could educate others about dōTERRA, but I still needed to get over my false belief that I didn't deserve to earn money by selling to my friends and family. Having a group setting of educating was less of a block for me. I had found my new hobby—and was paid like it was a hobby.

Back then, I didn't believe I was a leader. I was passionate to empower others, but I had a lot of false beliefs about myself that I allowed to cloud my vision of who I really was. The beautiful things about dōTERRA is it presents an opportunity to rewrite those false beliefs. I've taken the opportunity as it has come my way; I want to listen to what I'm to learn. I want to take those messages and apply them so it doesn't have to be pounded into me fifteen times. In reality, we all screw up, and it's better to learn a lesson the first time instead of the fifteenth time. One thing I've learned is, women sell everything. We sell how amazing our kids are, why we bought something, why we are doing something… So why not continue the trend and sell to others why you choose to use dōTERRA?

I hit a point in my dōTERRA business where I was creating an income, beyond just paying for my products, and I got there because of the business model of network marketing. "It's my business alone, but I'm not in it alone," I said. I had an upline who believed in a vision beyond what I was able to believe. Kierston Kirschbaum, my friend, and mentor, believed in me, and I began believing in myself until I made it (also known as "fake it till you make it!). The next level of belief was presented a few months later when Joey and I attended a convention. He looked at me and said "Let's build to Diamond."

"Do you know how much work and sacrifice that will be, as a mother of three young children, homeschooling, while you work 50 hours a week at your job?"

We agreed to the task at hand and focused our thoughts on "short-term sacrifice for a long-term reward."

While we were at that convention, I dreamt of traveling more, seeing more of the world. I had been to a couple of states, but now I wanted my travel opportunities to expand internationally—and now I travel all over the United States and internationally. Then I wondered, what would it look like if I were able to travel to these locations with my entire family so I can work and have my family with me, continue to educate others, support my teams, and see the world? It's all a belief! What if I told you the only thing holding you back from being exactly where you want to be in life is a belief? Opportunities will come your way. You will have a chance to grab them and learn and expand—or you can turn away and let them pass you by.

Before hitting Diamond, I recognized I had a false belief of who I would become if I had money. I was exposed to a powerful financial why and realized all the good I could do with acquiring financial freedom. Earlier in the month of March 2012, I shifted my false belief, and that month I hit Diamond. It was six months after our commitment, and I realized I could have accomplished this years sooner if I shifted out of the financial block sooner.

This is a journey, and the thoughts that lead you will make it what it is. You control your thoughts, or your thoughts control you. Love yourself unconditionally, and you'll see firsthand the power behind unconditional love. I wake up every morning and say to myself looking in the mirror at myself, "I am worthy, and my self-worth is in my Savior." Come up with your saying to say to yourself so you're putting your self-worth in something other than what others think of you, or in what you have. I know I'm going to keep building and keep growing. I've found—and will continue to find—amazing leaders who I'll get the chance to work with, because I believe it, and what you believe will manifest itself.

What would it be like if you could get rid of all your false beliefs? Know that you can. Give yourself permission to get rid of your false beliefs, beginning now. They are not real, and they are just building blocks in front of you that are holding you back from being your true self. Get rid of those and become your true self!

There's all sorts of false beliefs, and they can come from external sources. Others can judge you and they can try to put their false beliefs on you, whether they are judging themselves or you. When I feel others' judgments, filled with false beliefs coming my way, I mentally or even physically close my eyes and say, "This is not my junk." I envision myself pushing their junk away from myself.

It's easy for each of us to put our "junk" on others, and it's usually the ones we love the most. First, don't allow others to put their junk on you. And then give others permission to not take your junk when you try to throw it on them. The owner of the junk is the only one who can remedy and truly get rid of the junk. Don't judge others; all you're doing is throwing junk on them, and that just bogs their life down. Stop judging people. They are doing exactly what they need to be doing right when they're doing it. The moment you judge them, you are taking responsibility to teach them what, who, when, where, and why they need to be. Instead, let them own their junk, love them unconditionally, and allow the universe to be in charge, to teach them who they need to be. Do you really want that responsibility of perfectly teaching people out of their junk? I don't! Stop judging, hold gratitude, and love in abundance, in your heart. It works! What you'll find is a new transformation happens. The more you love yourself and others unconditionally, the less junk you're carrying around without judging them.

The most exciting part of building this business was having my husband join me as his full-time "job" as well. We have found an amazing dynamic of leadership for our business, through complementing and letting each others' natural talents shine. Together we are able to mentor a larger variety of individuals because of the personality traits we each hold. My very first opportunity to share my leadership style was at a dōTERRA Leadership Training. I talked about the importance of maximizing communication through speaking the language of others based on their personality as well as learning to work with different personalities to benefit all involved instead of resisting the natural ways of others.

Had I not been willing to get uncomfortable and try, sacrificing in increments of three to six months for the past two years, we would still be planning our life around work. Now we are a family of dad and mom, five kids, and a dog, planning our work around our life.

My current role with dōTERRA feels like some pretty big shoes to fill. I'm growing into them! I spontaneously coached a friend with this saying: "Own your shoes." You might have been given really big shoes, but I know you can fill them. Or maybe you want to step up into some bigger shoes, even if they flop around awkwardly at first. You'll fill them, and one day you'll run in them. Focus on you and what you need to do to get there. Believe in your purpose, and you'll find it.

Cachay Wyson loves to have fun, create beautiful things and passionately lives life to its fullest. She began her adult career as a Cosmetologist beautifying others on the outside. Shortly thereafter she met Joey Wyson, and married seven months later, in the Las Vegas, Nevada Temple. Eleven years later they now have five children. While raising a family she built a successful essential oil business, with the support of her husband. She specializes in educating others on the beauty that lies within them, to celebrate the natural strengths, and face our ineffective traits that hold us back from becoming our true selves. **Learn more:** *www.joeyandcachay.com.*

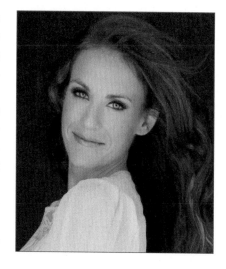

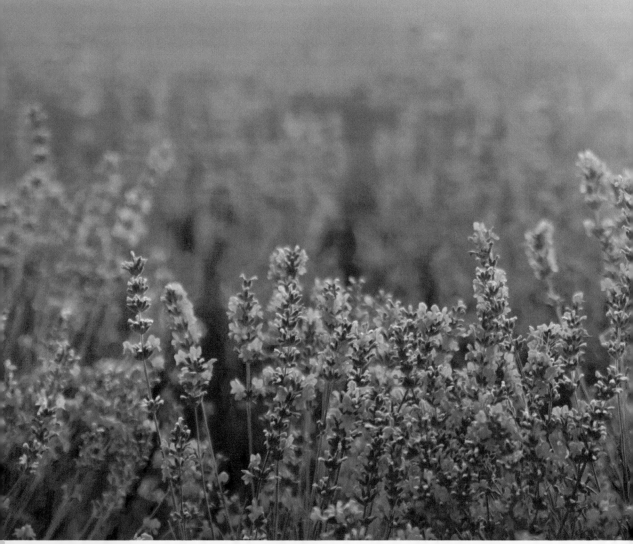

*The ground we walk on, the plants and creatures, the
clouds above constantly dissolving into new formations
—each gift of nature possessing its own radiant energy,
bound together by cosmic harmony.*

~Ruth Bernhard